TREATING CEREBRAL PALSY

To Dr. Harold Westlake, a pioneer in the development of speech and language therapy for the cerebral palsied.

Cover portrait of Harold Westlake by
John Wilson of Austin, Texas

FOR CLINICIANS BY CLINICIANS
Harris Winitz, Series Editor

This book, *Treating Cerebral Palsy*, is the fourth volume in the FOR CLINICIANS BY CLINICIANS series of texts on the diagnosis and clinical management of speech, language, and voice disorders. Each text provides a contemporary perspective on one major disorder or clinical area, and is designed for use in clinical methodology courses and continuing education programs. Authors have been selected who represent a broad spectrum of clinical interests and theoretical positions, but who hold the common belief that their viewpoints, experiences, and successes should be shared in order to provide a forum FOR CLINICIANS BY CLINICIANS.

Volumes already published in this series are *Treating Language Disorders, Treating Articulation Disorders,* and *Case Studies in Aphasia Rehabilitation.*

TREATING CEREBRAL PALSY

For Clinicians by Clinicians

Edited by
Eugene T. McDonald

8700 Shoal Creek Boulevard
Austin, Texas 78758

Printed in the United States of America

Library of Congress Cataloging in Publication Data

Treating cerebral palsy.

(For clinicians by clinicians)
Includes bibliographies and index.
1. Cerebral palsy—Treatment. I. McDonald,
Eugene T. (Eugene Thomas), 1916–   . II. Series.
[DNLM: 1. Cerebral palsy—therapy. WS 342 T784]
RC388.T67 1987   616.8'36   86-22568
ISBN 0-89079-141-4

pro·ed

8700 Shoal Creek Boulevard
Austin, Texas 78758

10 9 8 7 6 5 4 3   91

Contents

Contributors

Rona Alexander, PhD, CCC-SP
Private Practice
P.O. Box 26734
Wauwatosa, WI 53222

Faith Carlson, MS
The Rehabilitation Institute of
  Pittsburgh
6301 Northumberland Street
Pittsburgh, PA 15217

Jacqueline M. Doherty, RPT
Chief of Therapy
The Home of The Merciful Saviour
  for Crippled Children
4400 Baltimore Avenue
Philadephia, PA 19104

Robert H. Duckman, OD
Associate Professor of Optometry
State College of Optometry
State University of New York
100 East 24th Street
New York, NY 10010

Joseph L. French, EdD
Professor of Educational Psychology
The Pennsylvania State University
University Park, PA 16802

Eugene T. McDonald, EdD
Research Professor Emeritus,
  Speech Pathology
The Pennsylvania State University
University Park, PA 16802

Caroline R. Musselwhite, EdD
Communication Disorders
  Specialist
83 Keasler Road
Asheville, NC 28805

Lura G. Parker, MEd
Consultant, Early Childhood and
  Special Education
6315 Brook Lake Drive
Dallas, TX 75248

Bruce M. Siegenthaler, PhD
Research Professor Emeritus,
  Audiology
The Pennsylvania State University
University Park, PA 16802

Darcy Umphred, PhD
Partners in Learning Clinic
1639 Pacific Avenue
Rio Oso, CA 95674

Gregg C. Vanderheiden, PhD
Director, Trace Research and
  Development Center
University of Wisconsin
1500 Highland Avenue
Madison, WI 53705

Preface

To be effective, the treatment of cerebral palsy requires the coordinated efforts of several disciplines. When each discipline operates in isolation from the others, program quality is reduced. While each discipline has special knowledge and skills, there is a growing body of knowledge about cerebral palsy which must be understood by all members of the habilitation team because it is basic to all treatment and educational procedures. Communication among team members is facilitated when each discipline is aware of the basic concepts, treatment goals, and procedures of other disciplines.

Speech/language training cannot be divorced from physical therapy, occupational therapy, education, or any of the specialties concerned with habilitation of the person with cerebral palsy. Not only do these specialties have information needed by the speech/language pathologist, but they need information about speech/language pathology so they can further development and use of the child's communication skills.

From a book one can learn *about* cerebral palsy but all disciplines need *hands-on* experience to learn how to treat cerebral palsy. Speech/language pathologists must learn to use their eyes and hands as well as their ears. Such learning can occur only in practicums or through on-the-job training. This book is written to prepare students for further learning through the experience of working with persons who have cerebral palsy.

If a book about cerebral palsy were limited to only those statements which would be supported by experimental data and about which everyone agreed, it would be a small book. Unfortunately, while the number of scientific investigations is increasing, the body of experimentally derived data is small, especially in the area of treatment. Chapter authors have drawn on available research findings, but the major strength of this volume derives from the extensive clinical experience of the authors. It is inevitable that some procedures which have not yet been evaluated experimentally may be considered controversial. When based on an integration of science, clinical experience, and logical reasoning, such procedures have a place in clinical practice. We hope that this book will not only be used as a clinical manual but that it will also be used as a source of projects for researchers.

CHAPTER 1

Cerebral Palsy: Its Nature, Pathogenesis, and Management

Eugene T. McDonald

McDonald describes cerebral palsy as a complex condition resulting from a variety of etiological factors, manifesting a variety of neuromuscular symptoms and associated problems, and requiring a comprehensive program carried on by personnel from many disciplines.

1. *What do all persons with cerebral palsy have in common?*
2. *Several categories are used in describing or classifying cerebral palsy. What are the important features of each of the following categories: motor characteristics, topography, associated problems, and severity?*
3. *For each of the following periods, identify possible causes of cerebral palsy: prenatal, natal, and postnatal.*
4. *What are the elements of a comprehensive program designed to serve both individuals with cerebral palsy and the cerebral palsy population in general?*

INTRODUCTION

Anyone wanting to learn about cerebral palsy might ask three questions:

1. What is cerebral palsy?
2. What causes cerebral palsy?
3. What can be done about cerebral palsy?

These appear to be simple, straightforward questions but cerebral palsy is so complex that the questions call for elaborate discussions rather than simple, straightforward answers. In fact, with our present level of knowledge, complete answers cannot yet be given. Enough is known, however, to construct working answers which provide bases for diagnosis, assessment, treatment, and education.

WHAT IS CEREBRAL PALSY?

If all the persons who have cerebral palsy were brought together for examination, one would not need to be an expert in cerebral palsy to observe that the individuals differ markedly. They don't all look alike, act alike, or sound alike. Some would be so severely handicapped that they were totally dependent for even the most basic functions such as feeding and toileting. At the other extreme, some would be so mildly involved that their cerebral palsy would be noticed only by experts. They might not even be regarded as handicapped. Between these extremes, marked variability in symptomatology would be noted. Careful examination would reveal one common element—some type of *motor dysfunction resulting from* some type of *brain dysfunction*. Not all persons would exhibit the same motor symptoms nor would they all have the same brain pathology.

Definition

An answer to the question, "What is cerebral palsy?" must specify that there is an abnormality of motor function as a result of brain pathology. The role of brain dysfunction as the cause of abnormal motor function differentiates cerebral palsy from motor problems caused by spinal lesions such as poliomyelitis, spina bifida, and various paralyses associated with spinal cord injuries. Definitions of cerebral palsy also include the point that the brain dysfunction is the result of harmful events which occurred before, during, or soon after birth. This focus on time differentiates cerebral palsy from the motor problems caused by brain dysfunction associated with strokes or head injuries occurring later in life. Simply put, cerebral palsy is a condition characterized by motor dysfunction resulting from brain pathology which occurred before, during, or shortly after birth.

Such a simple definition, while accurate, is inadequate to answer the question, "What is cerebral palsy?" In fact, the term *cerebral palsy* is something of a misnomer. Pathologies resulting in the motor dysfunctions of cerebral palsy occur in parts of the brain other than the cerebrum. The term *palsy* is a synonym for *paralysis* which means a loss or impairment of motor function due to a lesion in the neural or the muscular mechanism. To the general public, however, the term *palsy* often suggests shaking and trembling—conditions not characteristic of all persons with cerebral palsy. Periodically groups interested in the problem have suggested that the term *cerebral palsy* be dropped; some authors and practitioners are using terms such as *neuromotor disability.* Use of cerebral palsy as a label is likely to continue because it has been used in fund raising, legislation, names of organizations, and facilities. It has too high a level of public awareness to be dropped. It is important, however, that professional workers using the term be mindful of its limitations.

To describe the nature of cerebral palsy, the simple definition must be expanded to include reference to what are often called "associated problems." Because of the central role the brain plays in cognitive processes and social-emotional behavior as well as in physical activities, impairment of intellectual functions, vision, and hearing are often found in cerebral palsy. Seizures and communication problems are common. Social-emotional development is affected. Severely involved individuals may have several of these problems; hence, persons with cerebral palsy are usually multiply handicapped. Learning disabilities, speech problems, vision, and hearing impairments often occur in individuals who do not have motor dysfunction associated with intracranial pathology. Such persons are not classified as cerebral palsied.

A broader definition might be worded as follows: Cerebral palsy is a multiply handicapping condition caused by brain abnormality resulting from maldevelopment or damage occurring before, during, or shortly after birth and characterized by motor dysfunction and a variety of associated problems. This definition has important implications for program planning because it focuses not only on the motor dysfunction but also on the associated problems which may be more limiting than the physical disability.

History of the Condition

Throughout history, children have been born with maldeveloped or injured brains. Among the sculptured monuments of Egypt and early stone carvings of Mexico are figures of individuals who appear to be cerebral palsied. One of the earliest descriptions of this condition was published by W. J. Little, an English physician, in 1843; in 1861 he elaborated on the condition which he referred to as "spastic rigidity." In addition to the motor dysfunction, Little noted other disorders such as intellectual impairment, seizures, and social-emotional problems. For many years, persons with motor dysfunction resulting from brain pathology of early origin were labeled spastic and considered to have Little's disease. The term *spastic* has lingered on as a generic label for the condition now known as cerebral palsy. In England and Australia, for example, organizations concerned with cerebral palsy are today called spastic societies.

During the second half of the 19th century, many physicians were interested in children with paralyses associated with intracranial pathology. There was speculation about the etiology of the condition and a growing awareness of the variety of physical manifestations. Some of the papers published during this period in the United States and Europe use the term *cerebral palsy* (e.g., Osler (1888) "The Cerebral Palsies of Children" and Sachs and Peterson (1890) "A Study of Cerebral Palsies of Early Life Based on an Analysis of One Hundred and Forty Cases"). Of special significance was Freud's book *Infantile Cerebral Paralysis* published in 1897 which influenced physicians of the time but was not widely known in America until translated in 1968.

The term *cerebral palsy* received wide professional acceptance when, in 1947, a group of physicians founded The American Academy for Cerebral Palsy. This group is now known as The American Academy for Cerebral Palsy and Developmental Medicine. Public awareness of the term has grown through the annual telethon and other activities of the United Cerebral Palsy Association.

Classifications of Cerebral Palsy

A review of the literature or of medical files reveals variations in classification systems. While three major categories—motor characteristics, topography, and severity—are widely used, the subcategories and nomenclature often differ. In 1954 the American Academy for Cerebral Palsy reviewed the variety of nomenclature and classifications in use. A system was proposed which included the following categories: physiologic (motor), topographic, etiologic, supplemental (associated problems), neuroanatomic, functional capacity (severity), and therapeutic. In this discussion of "What is cerebral palsy?" we will consider motor characteristics, topography, severity, and supplemental or associated problems. Etiology will be discussed in the section "What causes cerebral palsy?"

Motor Characteristics.   By definition, cerebral palsy is a motor disorder. The motor symptoms appear in a variety of forms, and several classification schemes are in use. The types described below are those suggested by the American Academy of Cerebral Palsy (AACP). The percentage given for each category is taken from a report analyzing 2,004 cases seen in a metropolitan (St. Louis, MO) cerebral palsy clinic (O'Reilly & Walentynowicz, 1981).

(1) *Spasticity.* The distinguishing feature of spasticity is a hyperactive stretch reflex. In normal function, the slight stretching of a muscle which occurs when its antagonist contracts stimulates the sensory endings in the neuromuscular spindles of the stretched muscle causing it to contract appropriately. A normal stretch reflex is essential for maintaining muscle tone and assists in the maintenance of posture. In spasticity, the response to stretching is exaggerated. During examinations this hyperactivity in spastics may be demonstrated when the examiner quickly extends the patient's flexed forearm causing a reflex contraction in the biceps which is being stretched during extension of the arm. Extension at the knee when the patellar tendon is struck and jerking movements of the foot in response to quick dorsiflexion are caused by hyperactive stretch reflexes. Spasticity often results in abnormal postures, contractures, and handicapping abnormalities of mobility. Spasticity is the most common type of cerebral palsy. Estimates vary, but most agree that more than half the cases fall in this category. In the St. Louis study, 62.8% were diagnosed as spastics.

(2) *Athetosis.* The distinguishing feature of athetosis is an abnormal amount of arrhythmic involuntary movement. An observer will note that, while reflexes are normal, performance of simple motor acts may be difficult or impossible because of the interference of uncontrollable involuntary movement. Diagnosticians agree that athetosis is the second most common type of cerebral palsy. In the St. Louis survey 11.7% were diagnosed as athetoids.

(3) *Rigidity.* The distinguishing neuromuscular characteristic of rigidity is resistance to flexion and extension movements resulting from continuous, simultaneous contraction of both the agonist and antagonist muscle groups. There are no hyperactive stretch reflexes or involuntary motions. Attempts to move a limb passively are often described as similar to trying to bend a lead pipe. In some persons the simultaneous contraction is intermittent, leading to a "cogwheeling" effect. Persons with rigidity are capable of only slow movements within a limited range. In the St. Louis survey 7.2% were classified as cases of rigidity.

(4) *Ataxia.* The distinguishing feature of ataxia is difficulty maintaining balance. Ataxia is usually not diagnosed until the child starts to walk. Typically, the feet are placed far apart and the feet are slapped down in taking steps. There is incoordination and clumsiness of movement. Reflexes are normal, but there may be hypotonia or muscular weakness. In the St. Louis study, 4.9% were diagnosed as ataxics.

(5) *Tremor.* The distinguishing characteristic of the tremor type of cerebral palsy is repetitive, rhythmic involuntary contractions of flexor and extensor muscles. These tremors may be intentional or nonintentional.

Intentional tremors are not present during rest but appear with voluntary or intended movement. Nonintentional tremors are present during rest and continue with intentional movement. Stretch reflexes are not hyperactive. In the St. Louis survey, 0.3% were of the tremor type.

Atonia. The term *atonia* means without or deficient in muscle tone. Some clinicians contend that atonia is not a type of cerebral palsy but rather one of the initial symptoms of a condition which later will be diagnosed as cerebral palsy—usually of the spastic or athetoid type (Bobath, 1966; Crothers & Paine, 1959; Denhoff & Robinault, 1960). In the St. Louis survey, 1.1% were diagnosed as cases of atonia.

Mixed. Careful examination of persons with cerebral palsy reveals that some exhibit combinations of neuromuscular characteristics. Use of this label varies widely. At one extreme Denhoff and Robinault (1960) suggest that this grouping need not be used often as the predominant motor symptoms determine the classification; whereas Crothers and Paine (1959) found frequent coexistence of spasticity and involuntary motion. They recommended frequent use of the term *mixed cerebral palsy.* The most common combination is spasticity in the lower extremities and athetosis in the arms and hands (Schleichkorn, 1983). In the St. Louis survey 12% of the cases were classified as mixed.

Those who work in the area of cerebral palsy must keep in mind the following points regarding classification on the basis of motor characteristics:

1. Nomenclature and classification are not uniform. Spasticity is universally used as a label. Some clinicians use the label *dyskinesia* in reference to athetosis, tremor, and rigidity. The athetoid type of cerebral palsy may be divided into subcategories such as tension, nontension, and dystonic.
2. It is often difficult to categorize the motor problems of infants and young children. What appears as a lack of muscle tone in infants may later appear in the form of athetosis or spasticity. The central nervous system continues to mature for several years after birth. Along with this development, the normally developing child becomes capable of increasingly complex and controlled movements. It is in trying to perform these motor acts that the motor symptoms of cerebral palsy are clarified.

Topography. In this context, *topography* refers to an anatomical region or special part of the body. In cerebral palsy classifications, the reference is to the number and location of limbs involved. The most common pattern is for the dyskinesias to affect all extremities, whereas spasticity appears in a variety of topographical forms. The four most common topographies are *hemiplegia, paraplegia, quadraplegia,* and *diplegia.* In hemiplegia, the most common type, one side of the body—either right or left—is involved. Only the legs are involved in paraplegia. In quadraplegia all four limbs are involved. In diplegia all four extremities are involved; however, the legs are involved primarily and there is only slight involvement of the arms. Involvement of one limb, monoplegia and of three limbs, triplegia is rare.

Topography of involvement has important implications for programming and eventual level of independence achieved. For example, paraplegics, with their good arm and hand function and good speech, can handle well most activities of daily living even though they may need aid in ambulation. Quadraplegics may remain dependent on others because poor control of their upper extremities precludes development of self-help skills.

Severity. The American Academy for Cerebral Palsy defined degree of severity in terms of functional capacity (Minear, 1956).

Class I—No practical limitation of activity
Class II—Slight to moderate limitation of activity
Class III—Moderate to great limitation of activity
Class IV—Unable to carry on any useful physical activity

This classification indicates the wide range of involvement; however, its usefulness is limited by the subjective meanings of "slight" and "moderate." Rusk (1977) proposed a classification based on competence in carrying out the basic self-help behaviors essential to everyday living, including communication.

Mild. A person with self-help skills adequate for caring for daily personal needs, who ambulates without appliances and has no speech problem. No treatment is needed.

Moderate. Self-help skills are inadequate, and the person may need special equipment for ambulation. Speech may be defective. Treatment of various types is needed.

Severe. Even with treatment and the use of adaptive equipment, the prognosis for developing self-help skills, ambulation, and functional speech is poor.

Associated Problems. The list of disorders associated with cerebral palsy is long. Some are the result of the same etiology as the motor dysfunction. Others, such as social-emotional problems, are secondary and result from environmental conditions created by the cerebral palsy. The associated problems will be covered more fully in subsequent chapters. The following brief discussion is included to further the consideration of classifications. It is not meaningful to cite the percentage of persons with cerebral palsy who exhibit the following disorders because the percentage would vary with the motor characteristics, topography, and severity.

Intellectual Impairment. The American Association on Mental Deficiency (1983) defined mental retardation as "significantly subaverage general intellectual functioning concurrently resulting in or associated with impairments in adaptive behavior and manifested during the developmental period." Many persons with cerebral palsy are described by this definition. Even though it is often difficult to determine whether the deficits in adaptive behavior can be attributed to motor dysfunction or intellectual impairment, it is clear that the distribution of intelligence differs from that of the general population. More persons are below average and fewer are in the average and above-average categories. There is a close relationship between incidence of mental retardation and the severity and topography of motor dysfunction. This is not to say, however, that all severe quadraplegics are intellectually impaired. Many are, but some demonstrate average and above-average intellectual ability. The question is often asked, "Is intellectual impairment caused by cerebral palsy?" The answer is "No, but mental retardation may be caused by the maldevelopment of or injury to the brain which also caused the cerebral palsy."

Sensory Dysfunction. All sensory modalities are vulnerable in cerebral palsy. Many of the etiological factors in cerebral palsy also cause visual disorders such as oculomotor defects, refractive errors and central processing problems. The incidence of hearing impairment has decreased since methods were developed to prevent erythroblastosis and rubella; however, infants with cerebral palsy are still at risk for sensorineural hearing loss. Also they are at risk for conductive loss because the combination of poor oropharyngeal motor control and poor alignment of the airway creates conditions conducive to development of middle ear infections. Body sensations, somesthesia, may be affected. Some children exhibit diminished tactile sensitivity, while others are hypersensitive to tactile stimulation. Body sensations associated with posture and movement (proprioception, kinesthesis, and vestibular motion) are often diminished or disordered.

Communication Problems. Children with moderate and severe cerebral palsy are at high risk for developing competence in communicating. Speech production is affected when the neuromuscular disorder extends to the speech mechanism. In severe cases the production of intelligible speech is impossible, and the use of communication aids such as language boards and minicomputers is limited because of poor upper-extremity control. Some children have central processing problems which interfere with language development.

Social-Emotional Complications. Many children with cerebral palsy are deprived of the interpersonal relationships and the personal achievements which contribute to positive social-emotional development. Initial bonding between infant and mother may be weak because the infant is difficult to feed and handle. The child's dependence on others interferes with development of a positive self-concept. Repeated failure in attempts to perform such simple tasks as feeding, toileting, and dressing result in low self-esteem. Some persons with severe neuromotor dysfunction settle into the role of passive recipients of care, often making little attempt to function at the level their degree of handicap would permit.

Educational Difficulties Several factors operate to create special educational problems for persons with cerebral palsy. The achievement of some, even with special programs, will be limited by the extent of their retardation. Problems with attention, memory, and perception interfere with learning. The handling of educational materials such as pencils and books is difficult for children with poor control of their arms and hands. Social-emotional factors may result in poor motivation, and sensory dysfunctions may interfere with the acquisition of knowledge and skills.

Seizure Disorders Among the causes of recurrent convulsions are congenital malformations of the brain and damage to the brain following hemorrhage or lack of oxygen (Baird, 1972). Since these factors figure prominently as causes of cerebral palsy, it is to be expected that many children with cerebral palsy will have some type of seizure. The most common type of seizure, grand mal, is characterized by a loss of consciousness. If standing or sitting, the child will fall over. There is a period of generalized stiffening followed by vigorous movements of the extremities. These attacks are usually followed by confusion and lethargy, and the child may fall asleep for as long as several hours. In petit mal seizures there is a momentary lapse of consciousness and the child briefly loses contact with the environment. Usually the eyes roll upward, the lids open and close rapidly, and the head nods rhythmically for a few seconds. There may be jerking of the body or limbs. Psychomotor seizures also occur in cerebral palsy. These are characterized by inappropriate or purposeless behavior lasting for a few minutes for which there is later no memory. Persons working with a child who has cerebral palsy might overlook petit mal or psychomotor seizures. The Epilepsy Foundation of America suggests that repeated occurrences of two or more of the following symptoms happening together and without variation may indicate a seizure disorder: staring spells resembling daydreaming, tic-like movements, rhythmic movements of the head, purposeless sounds and body movements, head dropping, lack of response, eyes rolling upward, chewing, and swallowing movements.

Physical Disability The child with cerebral palsy might have an orthopedic problem which any other child might have—clubfoot, congenital deformities of the spine, and so forth. These problems are not the result of cerebral palsy; however, the abnormal muscle tone associated with cerebral palsy may cause restricted joint motion in upper and lower extremities and may produce spinal deformities. One of the most common orthopedic problems is dislocation of one or both hips. The National Information Center for Handicapped Children and Youth reports that cerebral palsy accounts for a large portion of school–aged children with physical or health impairments.

WHAT CAUSES CEREBRAL PALSY?

Cerebral palsy may be the result of a multiplicity of causes. Whatever interferes with development of, or damages the brain may cause cerebral palsy. Events resulting in malfunction of the brain may occur during the prenatal, perinatal, or postnatal periods.

Prenatal

A brief review of prenatal development will help us understand why some children have cerebral palsy. Development begins when a sperm penetrates an ovum. Each sperm and each ovum contains 23 chromosomes. One of the 23 is the sex chromosome, and the remaining 22 are called *autosomes*. At conception, the chromosomes form 23 pairs; thus human beings have 46 chromosomes which carry all the information necessary to direct development from one cell to the highly complex arrangement of two hundred billion cells delivered as a baby approximately nine months later. On each chromosome are genes which control the function of cells and transmit hereditary traits. Thus a child might inherit blue or brown eyes, be tall or short, have black, white, yellow or, perhaps, as in albinism, a form of birth defect, no coloring matter in the skin. The structure of genes is complex and many factors may cause mistakes in the chemical coding within a gene. Approximately 200 types of birth defects are known to be caused by defective genes. Because genes are paired at conception—one from the mother and one from the father—a person might have a defective (recessive) gene that does not cause a defect because it is paired with a normal (dominant) gene. Such a person is called a *carrier*. If two carriers of the same recessive gene mate, there is one chance in four that the child will inherit both abnormal genes and have a birth defect. In addition to autosomal recessive inheritance as a cause of birth defects, there are instances (e.g., Huntington's chorea) where one abnormal gene, called an *autosomal dominant*, is sufficient for expression of the trait. Denhoff and Robinault (1960) estimated that at least 10% of cerebral palsy is the result of hereditary factors.

Development proceeds rapidly after the sperm enters the ovum. Within a few hours, the cell containing chromosomes from mother and father divides to become two cells which divide to become four cells, the four become eight, and so on. Some cells have developed characteristics different from the others by the time the cell mass contains 32 cells. The cells group to form a hollow sphere known as a *morula* which consists of two cavities separated by a plate of cells, the embryonic disc, from which the new individual develops. The outer cells of the morula become part of the placenta, a temporary organ which anchors the fetus to the uterus and through which the fetus receives oxygen and nourishment and discharges wastes. The cellular wall of the cavity above the embryonic disc forms the fluid-filled amniotic sac in which the fetus floats. The lower cavity, a yolk sac, disappears about 10 weeks after conception. From the ectoderm, the upper layer of cells on the embryonic disc, the skin and nervous system develop. From the lower layer, the endoderm, develops the lining of the digestive and respiratory tracts. From the middle layer, mesoderm, muscle, bones, and connective tissue develop.

Development is a biochemical process. All living organisms function as complex biochemical systems from conception to death. During human development, body parts are formed by orderly sequences of cell divisions, cell growth, cell differentiation, and cell rearrangement—all of which occur in response to precisely timed chemical reactions. Anything that disrupts the orderly sequence of complex chemical reactions may result in a birth defect such as cerebral palsy.

For our study of cerebral palsy, development of the central nervous system is of special interest. About three weeks after conception, the upper layer of cells of the embryonic disc thickens to form the neural plate. The edges of this flat plate fold to form the neural tube which initially is open on both ends. This tunnel becomes the central canal and ventricles around which the brain and spinal cord develop. The brain develops from the inside out, and overall, development recapitulates human evolutionary development. Beginning as three swellings at the front of the tube, the forebrain, midbrain, and hindbrain develop. The forebrain divides into the telencephalon (endbrain) and diencephalon (throughbrain). The midbrain, or mesencephalon (middle brain) does not subdivide. The hindbrain divides into the metencephalon (afterbrain) and the myelencephalon (marrow brain). Figure 1.1 shows how several major parts of the mature brain evolve from the embryonic neural tube.

By the end of the second month, which marks the end of the embryonic period and beginning of the fetal period, the brain and spinal cord resemble that of the adult in arrangement and form. Movement, which began during the second month, becomes more vigorous and complex during the third month. The fetus can kick, pivot, and twist; move the thumb in opposition to the fingers; open the mouth; swallow, inhale, and exhale. Curling the toes, bending the wrist, and making a fist occur (Apgar & Beck, 1974). Clearly the first trimester is a period of rapid neuromotor development. Although the gross structures of the brain are in place, important intrinsic differentiations have not yet taken place, especially in the neocortex

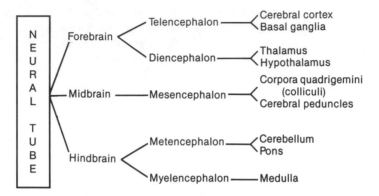

Figure 1.1. Brain development.

of the telencephalon. Development continues throughout the fetal period. Cells multiply, dendrites grow, and synapses form. There is a spurt in brain growth beginning in the third trimester and continuing into the second year. Sensory functions also develop prenatally. Sensory discriminations have been demonstrated in the gustatory, olfactory, and auditory modalities a few hours after birth. The newborn's ability to carry out cross-modal functions is demonstrated by the observation that babies only a few days old will stick out their tongue in imitation of an adult. These infants process information from visual stimulation to form a motor command to tongue musculature.

This brief and simplified description of prenatal neuromotor development points up the vulnerability of the rapidly developing, highly complex structures comprising the brain. Earlier we noted that abnormal genes may carry a blueprint for abnormal development. Normal development may be disrupted by anything that interferes with the biochemistry of development or with the supply of oxygen and nutrients. Some disruptions result in termination of development followed by miscarriage or stillbirth. Parts of the brain might fail to develop or, after development, atrophy. Resulting neuromotor dysfunction may range from the hard neurologic signs present in cerebral palsy to the so-called "soft" signs some clinicians associate with learning disabilities. Some maternal infections (e.g., rubella, cytomegalovirus, toxoplasmosis, herpes) and incompatibility between fetal and maternal blood, especially for the Rh factor, may adversely affect the brain of the fetus. A variety of factors (e.g., defects in the placenta or umbilical cord) may interfere with brain's oxygenation. Prenatal cerebral hemorrhage might be associated with toxemia of pregnancy. Maternal metabolic disorders such as diabetes can have adverse effects on the prenatal brain. Chronic maternal alcoholism and perhaps even moderate ingestion of alcohol may cause brain damage. Smoking and the use of drugs—even some prescription drugs—during pregnancy are now suspect as causative agents in brain dysfunction.

Perinatal

Intrauterine development began within a single cell so small as to be barely visible to the unaided eye. It would take about 175 arranged in a row to make an inch. For approximately nine months the mother has been a hospitable host to this new being which now possesses 200 billion cells, and on the average is 20 inches long and weighs 7¼ pounds. The time to be born has arrived.

The mother, no longer a hospitable host, initiates vigorous actions to expel the fetus. Contractions of uterine muscles force the baby downward through the birth canal—a trip which has been described as the most hazardous journey any individual will ever make. Delivery is through an opening in the bony pelvic girdle which must widen to permit the baby's passage. During the birth process the amniotic sac ruptures, releasing the fluid which provided protection for the fetus in a warm and constant temperature. The infant must pass, usually head first, through the narrow confines of the birth canal without this protection. Fortunately at this stage of development the bones of the skull are not rigidly joined together, allowing some displacement without fracturing bones or damaging underlying brain tissues. Most infants make their way through the birth canal with nothing more than a few bruises. They quickly gasp for breath and utter a cry. With the cutting of the now useless umbilical cord, the infant is no longer biologically attached to the mother. It is now time to establish the psychosocial attachments which will be discussed in a later chapter.

Not all births are uneventful. Sometimes the trauma associated with difficult labor or the sudden pressure changes associated with precipitate delivery cause intracranial hemorrhaging with resultant brain damage. The list of factors which can cause anoxia and damage brain cells includes respiratory obstructions, collapsed lungs, premature separation of or abnormal position of the placenta, and deliveries in which emergence of the head is delayed. Pain-relieving medications administered to the mother quickly enter the circulatory system of the fetus and may depress neo-natal respiratory function. In difficult deliveries, obstetric intervention may result in brain damage. Children born prematurely are at high risk for cerebral palsy.

Postnatal

We noted earlier that cerebral palsy is the result of brain pathology which occurred before (prenatal), during (perinatal) or shortly after (postnatal) birth. *How long* after birth is not a definitely defined period. A child who, after birth, has enjoyed a period of normalcy before development was interrupted by brain damage has a more mature nervous system than a newborn. Rapid acquisition of knowledge and skills begins at birth. In all areas—physical, cognitive and social-emotional—children advance each day. Each advance produces neuronal patterns which are not completely destroyed by postnatal trauma; hence, the symptomatology depends on how much the child had learned before the brain was damaged.

The causes of postnatal brain trauma are many. Fractures of the skull or penetrating head wounds may result from accidents. Infections such as meningitis, encephalitis, and brain abscesses may occur during childhood as well as later in life. Cerebral hemorrhage might result from the rupture of a congenital aneurysm of a blood vessel in the brain. Brain tumors, if permitted to expand, may damage brain cells as may surgical removal of the neoplasm. Asphyxia with lowered oxygen level may occur in near drowning, strangulation, or smoke inhalation. Neurotoxins such as lead may damage the brain.

What causes cerebral palsy? We have not attempted to list all the causes. Rather, we have suggested various kinds of etiological factors which interfere with development or injure developed brain cells. These factors alter the chemistry of, reduce the oxygen supply to, or mechanically damage brain cells.

WHAT CAN BE DONE ABOUT CEREBRAL PALSY?

This question must be answered on two levels: What can be done for the individual with cerebral palsy? What can be done about the problem of cerebral palsy in general? Some communities and some agencies prefer to concentrate their financial resources and personal efforts on providing direct services to the person handicapped by cerebral palsy. Such a philosophy is short sighted because many of the individual's needs can be approached only through programs which address the general problem of cerebral palsy. For example, public education, while not a direct service, is essential. Information about cerebral palsy must be widespread to generate adequate public support of treatment programs and research and to develop acceptance of disabled persons as full members of society. Financial support of research is not a direct service, but research produces knowledge which may be applied to an individual's problems. A comprehensive program of broad scope is required. It must include efforts directed to the general problems which transcend the immediate needs of the individual and also provide, at the state-of-the-art level, those direct services needed by the individual. A comprehensive program would include the following:

Public Education

Unless aroused, the general public tends to be apathetic regarding the needs of persons with handicaps. In fact many people appear to be afraid of disabled persons and are uncomfortable in their presence. In the past, most public education programs have been linked with fund raising activities by the National Easter Seal Society and United Cerebral Palsy Associations. Recently the National Information Center for Handicapped Children and Youth was established to answer questions, sponsor workshops, publish newsletters, and provide educational materials. Increasingly persons with handicaps—including cerebral palsy—are speaking out and assuming advocacy roles. A climate of understanding and acceptance is developing slowly. Architectural barriers are coming down, facilities for independent living are increasing, and more persons with cerebral palsy are finding employment.

Prevention

Because of the multiplicity of causes, all cerebral palsy cannot be prevented; however, a number of causes can now be controlled. An inoculation is available which prevents rubella. Medical treatments now in use have essentially eliminated the cerebral palsy formerly caused by Rh incompatibility. Infectious diseases such as meningitis and encephalitis now respond to treatment before causing brain damage. Changes in prenatal care and obstetric management have reduced the risk of brain damage. Prevention of cerebral palsy of unknown origin, usually classified as idiopathic, and postnatal trauma remain a challenge (O'Reilly & Walentynowicz, 1981).

Approximately 50% fewer babies were born with cerebral palsy in 1978 than in 1958 according to a report of the United Cerebral Palsy Research and Educational Foundation (Richmond, 1978). The St. Louis study reported a decreasing incidence in cerebral palsy, which the authors attributed to improved prenatal and perinatal care. They point out, however, that their figures may also reflect the decline in birth rate which began in the late 1950s. The extent of the influence of preventative measures on the incidence and prevalence of cerebral palsy is unclear. Several studies cited by Kiely, Paneth, Stein, Susser (1981) indicate an overall downward trend, but they conclude ". . . the notion of a steady reduction in cerebral palsy prevalence rates corresponding to improved neonatal care is not sustained by the available evidence" (pp. 533–538).

Case Finding, Diagnosis, and Evaluation

Although reports of medical investigations of cerebral palsy began appearing in the literature during the 1850s, it was almost 100 years before treatment programs were described. At that time cerebral palsy was often not recognized until the child had failed to learn to walk. Barsch (1968) reported that two-thirds of the children attending a cerebral palsy clinic in Milwaukee had received a diagnosis of cerebral palsy between birth and one year. A diagnosis of cerebral palsy had been made for 88% by age two. Development of procedures for assessing the status of newborns and young infants has led to early identification of children at risk for neuro-motor and other developmental disabilities. Assessment and evaluation of infants at risk now begins in the newborn nursery and continues in other settings as the infant matures. Researchers and clinicians are now assessing the child's cognitive and affective status as well as the physical condition. Diagnosis does not end with the determination that a child has cerebral palsy. Causes of the symptoms of associated problems which appear must be determined. Periodic evaluations are required to provide bases for treatment and educational programs.

Treatment and Education

Diagnostic and evaluative studies are not ends in themselves. A comprehensive program must include the therapeutic procedures indicated by these studies and educational programs appropriate to the child's needs and abilities.

Children with cerebral palsy need routine medical care for the usual childhood health problems, and many need attention for special problems such as seizures, visual disorders, and orthopedic problems. Because of feeding difficulties, regular dental care is essential to maintain good oral hygiene. Most will at some time require physical therapy, occupational therapy, and speech-language therapy. Infant stimulation programs have evolved in response to increased awareness of the importance of stimulation to all areas of development. Education integrated with the various therapies now begins long before children reach school age. A growing number of persons with cerebral palsy continue their education through high school and college.

Counseling

It is natural that having a child with cerebral palsy in the family will create emotional stresses for the parents, siblings, and other family members. Parents often need help in recognizing and handling their feelings. There is growing awareness that social-emotional development is adversely affected by cerebral palsy (Gliedman & Roth, 1980). Many young adults with cerebral palsy are not prepared to cope with the emotional problems of everyday living. Psychological adjustment problems of parents and the handicapped child may begin at the time of the child's birth. Each stage of development brings additional stresses. Crisis-oriented counseling is not the answer. Counseling should be available on a continuing basis. Counselors (a social worker, psychologist, or other trained person) should be provided as members of the rehabilitation team.

Recreation

Play for children and recreation for adults are often regarded as frivolous, leisure time activities. Behavioral scientists now recognize that play contributes to cognitive development as well as to the physical and emotional health of children (Chance, 1979). For the adolescent and adult, recreational activities afford opportunities for socializing which contribute to good mental health. Year-round appropriate recreational activities should be provided at each age level for persons with cerebral palsy.

Employment

It is difficult for persons with severe motor dysfunction to find gainful employment, although technological advances are now creating more vocational opportunities. Persons with cerebral palsy should have access to vocational guidance, training, and job placement services including sheltered workshop programs for those unable to qualify for competitive employment.

Appropriate Living Arrangements

Most persons with cerebral palsy live with their parents. While there are advantages to this arrangement, it is not always possible or desirable for the handicapped person to live at home with members of the family. Parents eventually become physically unable to provide the care required by a person whose condition is severe and, of course, arrangements for care must be made for when the parents are no longer alive. Many young adults with cerebral palsy prefer to live away from home and have their needs met by personal care attendants rather than parents. The trend is toward small community living arrangements rather than large residential institutions. There is a great need for such facilities; however, it is likely that there will also be a continuing need for some larger, perhaps state operated, residential facilities. When the person with severe cerebral palsy continues to live at home, parents sometimes need time off, but they can't leave their child alone. There is a need for facilities where the child—or adult—can live temporarily not only in a time of emergency but periodically, to give parents relief from the stress of constant care.

Research

Investigation of problems related to cerebral palsy is supported by several agencies such as the National Institute of Health, U.S. Department of Education, United Cerebral Palsy Research and Education Foundation, and the National Easter Seal Society. Even with these ongoing efforts many crucial problems are not receiving attention. Every aspect of cerebral palsy has many unanswered questions. There are as yet unknown causes, and how some known causes operate is not understood. Diagnostic procedures and preventive measures must be developed and evaluated. Many treatment procedures in every discipline are largely based on theory with little empirical support. Scientific investigation of the efficacy of therapeutic and educational practices is lacking. Only a few cerebral palsy centers regard research as an essential component of their programs. It is clear that our current approaches fall short of helping cerebral palsied persons reach their highest functional level. New knowledge is needed. The development of knowledge through research is slow, painstaking, and expensive—there is no alternative.

Personnel Training

Recruitment and training of the professional, student, and volunteer lay personnel needed in all areas of a comprehensive program must be conducted in an organized manner.

Funding and Financial Aid

Both the general program and the direct services have a continuing need for financial support. Fund raising and financial aid are important components of a comprehensive approach to addressing the problems of cerebral palsy. The nationwide annual appeals of the National Easter Seal Society and the United Cerebral Palsy Associations raise money. Through several government agencies, money from taxes is directed to cerebral palsy. Eligible disabled persons may receive aid through the Social Security Administration. At the local level, some aid is available through such fund raising agencies as United Way.

CONCLUSION

This section addressed the question, "What can be done about cerebral palsy?" It is also important to consider, "What can't be done about cerebral palsy?" We must remember that cerebral palsy is an irreversible condition. While a comprehensive program will help many develop ambulation, communication skills, and competence in carrying out the activities of daily living, some individuals will remain dependent on other people for assistance with even the most basic of everyday activities. A comprehensive program can facilitate the care of those who cannot care for themselves and help others learn to function with varying degrees of independence even though their manner of functioning is not normal.

REFERENCES

Apgar, V., & Beck, J. (1974). *Is my baby all right?* New York: Simon and Schuster (Pocket Book Edition).

Baird, H. W. (1972). *The child with convulsions.* New York: Grune and Stratton.

Barsch, R. H. (1968). *The parent of the handicapped child.* Springfield, IL: Charles C Thomas.

Bobath, K. (1966). *The motor deficits in patients with cerebral palsy.* Levenham, England: Spastic International Medical Publications.

Chance, P. (1979). *Learning through play.* New York: Garden Press.

Crothers, B., & Paine, R. (1959). *The natural history of cerebral palsy.* Cambridge: Harvard University Press.

Denhoff, E., & Robinault, I. (1960). *Cerebral palsy and related disorders.* New York: McGraw Hill.

Freud, S. (1968). *Infantile cerebral paralysis* (L. A. Russin, Trans.). Coral Gables: University of Miami Press. (Original work published 1897)

Gliedman, J., & Roth, W. (1980). *The unexpected minority.* New York: Harcourt, Brace, Jovanovich.

Grossman, H. G. (1983). *Classification in mental retardation.* Washington, DC: American Association on Mental Deficiency.

Kiely, J. L, Paneth, N., Stein, Z., & Susser, M. (1981). Cerebral palsy and newborn care: Part I. Secular trends in cerebral palsy. *Developmental Medicine and Child Neurology, 23,* 533–538.

Little, W. J. (1843). Course of lectures on deformation of the human frame. *Lancet, 1,* 318.

Little, W. J. (1861). On the influence of abnormal parturition, difficult labor, premature birth, and asphyxia neonatorium, on the mental and physical condition of the child, especially in relation to deformities. *Lancet, 2,* 378–380.

Minear, W. L. (1956). A classification of cerebral palsy. *Pediatrics, 28,* 841–852.

O'Reilly, D. E., & Walentynowicz, J. E. (1981). Etiological factors in cerebral palsy: An historical review. *Developmental Medicine and Child Neurology, 23,* 633–642.

Osler, W. (1888). The cerebral palsies of children. *Medical News.*

Richmond, J. B. (1978). *Investing in our children.* Research Report. New York: United Cerebral Research and Educational Foundation.

Rusk, H. (1977). *Rehabilitation medicine* (4th ed.). St. Louis: C. V. Mosby.

Sachs, B., & Peterson, S. (May, 1980). A study of cerebral palsies in early life based on an analysis of 140 cases. *Journal of Nervous Diseases.*

Schleichkorn, J. (1983). *Coping with cerebral palsy.* Austin, TX: PRO-ED.

CHAPTER 2

Neurophysiologic Bases of Modern Treatment Procedures

Darcy A. Umphred

Umphred notes that several currently popular approaches to the treatment of cerebral palsy base their rationale and procedures on interpretation of central nervous system (CNS) functioning. She contends that effective use of any approach requires an understanding of the neurophysiologic and neuropsychologic principles on which the technique is based and how the child receives, processes, and responds to stimulation.

1. *What is the basic neuronal arrangement by which the organism receives, processes, and responds to internal and external stimuli?*
2. *The neurophysiologic process of facilitation and inhibition are frequently used in the treatment of cerebral palsy. How do facilitation and inhibition occur in the CNS? Make a list of the stimuli and techniques which Umphred describes as facilitating and those which she describes as inhibiting.*
3. *What is meant by "encephalization"? What is the significance of encephalization for normal development and for the treatment of cerebral palsy?*
4. *Some therapies employ various types of sensory stimulation for a number of reasons such as altering motor responses and heightening alertness. What are the sensory systems, how are they stimulated, and how might such stimulation be employed in the treatment of cerebral palsy?*
5. *How does the motor system function in producing movement and in maintaining posture, and how do posture and movement interact in the production of speech?*

INTRODUCTION

Review of the early writings on the education and treatment of children with cerebral palsy suggests that neither the neurophysiologic character of the disorder nor the neurophysiologic basis of development and learning received adequate consideration. In part, this was because at that time, information about neurophysiologic processes was elementary and not sufficiently organized to provide a scientific basis for treatment and education. Techniques based largely on practical experience sometimes proved to be inappropriate, ineffective and, at times, counterproductive. There is now a large, and growing, body of neurophysiologic knowledge which has important implications for everyone who works with cerebral palsied children.

Cerebral palsy (CP) represents a variety of clinical problems with overlapping complexities. Categorization of the types of cerebral palsy leads to additional confusion because a single child may move from one diagnostic category to another during development of the CNS. The specific neuropathology leading to the nonprogressive neurological deficits of spasticity, athetosis, and ataxia have been traced primarily to ischemic and/or hypoxic insults to the CNS while in utero, during birth, or shortly thereafter (Coleman, 1981; Volpe, 1981; Volpe & Koenigsberger, 1981). The span of time after birth over which the diagnosis may be applied leads to even more controversy and confusion. The American Academy for Cerebral Palsy states that any child below age five who has a neuromotor problem resulting from a brain insult may be classified as cerebral palsied. Others use the limit of three years of age (Vining, 1976). Once the age limit has extended beyond birth or shortly thereafter, overlap with traumatic brain injury, near drownings, brain infections, seizure disorders, and metabolic imbalances causes confusion in identifying specific diagnosis, lesion sites, and subsequent neuromotor dysfunction. Understanding the organization of the CNS, the effect of myelination and maturation (Yakovleo & Lecours, 1967) and thus susceptibility of the CNS to insult at various stages of development facilitates comprehension of the magnitude of the problems encountered by a child with cerebral palsy. It is outside the scope of this chapter to discuss the neuropathology and neurological sequelae resulting from specific lesions within the CNS, and the reader is referred to additional sources (Coleman, 1981; Ito, 1979; Page & Wigglesworth, 1979). This chapter will discuss the normal organizational structure of the CNS, the input (sensory) systems providing information about the environment surrounding the child, the output (motor) systems available to the child leading to control over self.

Because the function of the CNS is to receive, assimilate, and act on information, some treatment approaches try to correct existing deficits. They tend to focus on the inherent correlation between normal sequential behavior development (Fiorentino, 1981; Illingsworth, 1980), inherent functioning of the CNS (Pribram, 1971), plasticity of the immature brain (Held, 1965), and the potential of the human mind to learn. To use these approaches effectively, the clinician must understand normal functioning of the neuromechanism. Without this knowledge the clinician often assumes that once a lesion exists, the specific function of that component of the CNS has been lost. Thus, teaching compensatory strategies which focus on development of other areas within the CNS may be the only treatment procedure available. Unfortunately for both the child and the clinician, this philosophy may then limit the scope of therapy, the expectations placed on the child, and ultimately the freedom available to the child to interact and control the environment. For example, many CP children lack adequate postural control of the trunk, neck, and oral-motor system. This lack of stabilization prevents development of normal respiration, feeding, and eventual speech production. If a therapist assumes that the postural deficit is irreversible, then a compensatory strategy for expressive communication must be taught to the child. On the other hand, a therapist who is aware of (a) the normal behavioral sequences which lead to postural development of the proximal musculature, (b) the normal neurophysiological systems involved in the production of that control, and (c) the sensory systems vital to providing input to facilitate postural development, can try to create a treatment program which facilitates good postural development and provides the motor mechanism for control over speech production. If treatment is successful, the child then has the option of using either speech or a compensatory strategy to communicate.

ORGANIZATION AND STRUCTURE OF THE CNS

The role of the CNS is to process information in an orderly fashion, enabling the organism to maintain internal homeostasis and to adapt to the world in a functional manner. The specific neurophysiology and its neuroanatomical basis which explain how homeostasis is obtained or how information is accepted, processed, and acted upon can be baffling to the basic neuroscientist. Viewed as a whole, the brain is a maze of circuits, on-off switches, receiving centers, generators, transmitters, and communication networks. This system seems to go everywhere, do everything, and somehow summate all available information into a meaningful whole in order to direct purposeful activity, allowing the individual to control the environment on a moment-to-moment basis.

An elementary understanding of the structure and function of the CNS may be gained by studying block diagrams in which each block represents a component of the system. Starting with a simple model, blocks may be added to represent increasingly complex structure and function.

Neurons

Three types of neurons make up the basic structure and function of the CNS: (a) afferent (sensory) neurons which receive information from internal structures and the external environment, (b) motor (efferent) neurons which innervate smooth and skeletal muscle in order to carry out the instructions of the CNS, and (c) interneurons which process the information received as input in order to communicate the desired response to the motor neuron (Figure 2.1). The complexity of the CNS is based on these interneurons. Yet, in themselves, their function is limited. They either facilitate (encourage the passage of information to the next neuron) or inhibit (suppress the passage of information to the next neuron).

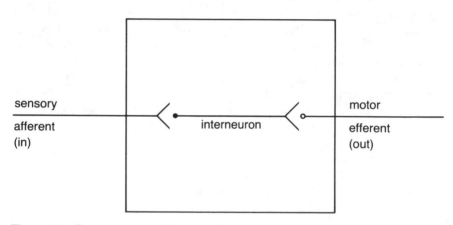

Figure 2.1.   Basic structure of the central nervous system.

Interneuronal Connections

As additional segments are added to the original model, a variety of potential interneuronal synaptic connections can be identified (Figure 2.2). With the introduction of segmental units, a basic spinal cord structure has been created. These structures would correspond to the long chain reflex arcs inherent to the human spinal system. A pattern of withdrawal to a noxious stimulus illustrates the behavioral component of the neuroanatomical system. As a stimulus enters one level (for example, segment 2 in Figure 2.2), it facilitates an interneuron which ascends and descends to other segments (projection interneuron) in order to recruit additional motor neurons to carry out a specific, preprogrammed, generalized response.

Through the use of these projection interneurons, a variety of combinations of facilitory and inhibitory influences can be established. If the

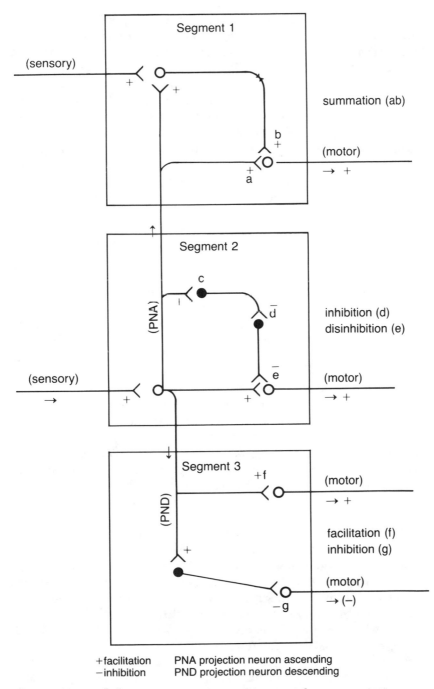

Figure 2.2. Interneuronal connections in a multisegmental nervous system.

ascending projection establishes a neuronal connection (synapse) with a motor neuron at a higher level as well as with other interneurons which facilitate that motor neuron, then summation of input occurs (Figure 2.2, 1a and b). If the interneuron facilitates an inhibitory neuron, it will tend to stop the flow of information at the next synaptic junction (Figure 2.2, 2d). If that inhibitory neuron synapses on another inhibitory neuron, (Figure 2.2, 2e) it will stop the second neuron from inhibiting at the synapse. This results in facilitation or lack of inhibition, a state referred to as *disinhibition*. To go one step farther, if the internuncial sends a facilitory collateral to one motor neuron (Figure 2.2, 3f) while facilitating an inhibitory interneuron going to an antagonistic motor neuron (Figure 2.2, 3g) then the potential for reciprocal organization of movement has been established.

Centralized Integration Center

To further control and modify the existing reflex loops found in the spinal system, a centralized integration center is needed (Figure 2.3). With this new center, sensory information not only affects the lower segmental portions of the CNS, it is also sent to higher centers for further processing. The central receiving area processes the data, stores it for future reference, and sends coded information back to the motor system in order to further refine and control the output or adaptation process of the organism.

Multiple Central Processing Centers

The human CNS has developed far beyond the simple organizational structure illustrated in Figure 2.2 as well as that shown in Figure 2.3. In a process called *encephalization*, centralized processing centers have been added, each building upon the next and thus adding further integration to the CNS. Encephalization has led to our unique ability to control, modify, and integrate multiple sensory inputs both simultaneously and successively. Creation of each new higher level processing center did not occur randomly; rather, the addition of new components has added to the control and modification of lower centers.

The design of the CNS is efficient and seems to be based on the underlying structural relationship. When analyzing the hierarchical relationship of structure and function within the CNS, a therapist can often determine which system naturally controls and modifies other systems. The following example illustrates how such an analysis may be used in planning treatment for a cerebral palsied child. Some severely involved children, when lying supine, exhibit strong extensor patterns causing the back to be arched. Strong extension tends to pull the jaw open, limit diaphragmatic excursion, forcefully pull the tongue into the back of the mouth, and inhibit swallowing due to the head positioning and lack of flexion. Knowing that the tonic labyrinthine reflex (TLR) is eliciting this

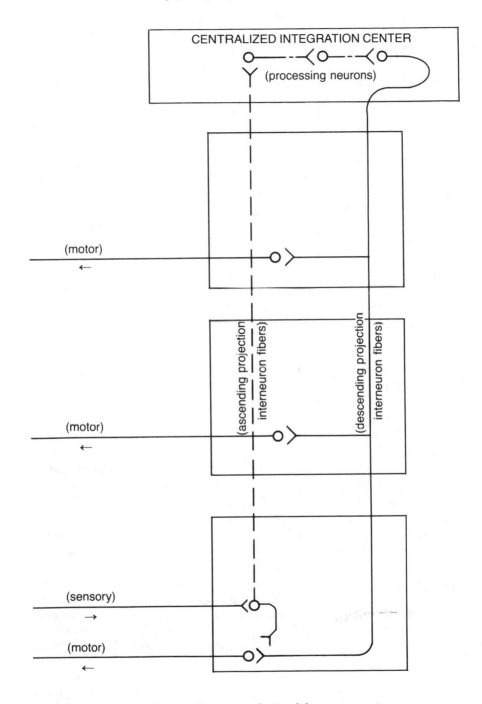

Figure 2.3. Projection fibers leading to complexity of the nervous system.

pattern and that it is processed in the lower brainstem—the medulla level of the CNS (Figure 2.4)—helps the clinician analyze how to inhibit the undesirable patterns and facilitate better respiratory, neck, and oral-motor control. Knowing that labyrinthine righting (LR) of the head, integrated at the collicular or midbrain level (Figure 2.4e)(Fiorentino, 1981), directly controls and modifies the influence of the TLR, immediately identifies treatment strategies. The clinician who knows that labyrinthine righting and optic righting of the head are optimally facilitated in vertical and the TLR maximally inhibited, and that flexion inhibits extension, has already identified a starting point. Positioning the child in a sitting position with limbs and trunk in a flexor pattern and the head vertical or slightly tipped backward should encourage neck flexion by eliciting both the LR and the stretch reflex. The flexor pattern should be facilitated if better respiratory, neck, and oral motor control is the goal.

The direction of treatment can vary, but the clinician has begun treatment using those central processing centers which most efficiently alter the undesired motor responses of excessive extensions. Using cognitive control centers to do the same job would require the child to expend much more energy—and might never be accomplished. To bypass the normal integration of the TLR by optic and labyrinthine righting of the head and demand, instead, that the child try to swallow or control the tongue placement, or even to suggest beginning encouragement of speech patterns, is most likely doomed to failure and frustration on the part of both the child and the clinician.

Central Nervous System Structures and Their Functions

The central nervous system consists of the spinal cord and the brain.

Spinal Cord. The spinal cord is the lowest segment of the central nervous system. It is made up of 31 segments which extend from the lower back (coccygeal-sacral region) to the upper neck (cervical region). Exteroceptive (cutaneous) and proprioceptive (joint, muscle spindle, tendon) afferent input from the lower extremities, trunk, upper extremities, and neck region enter the CNS at the spinal level. Efferent (motor) neurons going to the same body segments leave the nervous system at appropriate levels within the spinal segments. Stimuli coming from within the body—which tell higher centers about hunger, pain, temperature, etc.—also enter the CNS at many segmental areas of the spinal cord.

Afferents entering the spinal system provide information to higher centers about the external and internal environment. While multiple interneuronal projections ascend to higher integrative centers, a large number of collaterals and interneurons remain within the spinal segment, creating reflex loops that stimulate neurons at more than one segment within the spinal system. Some of the reflex patterns processed at the

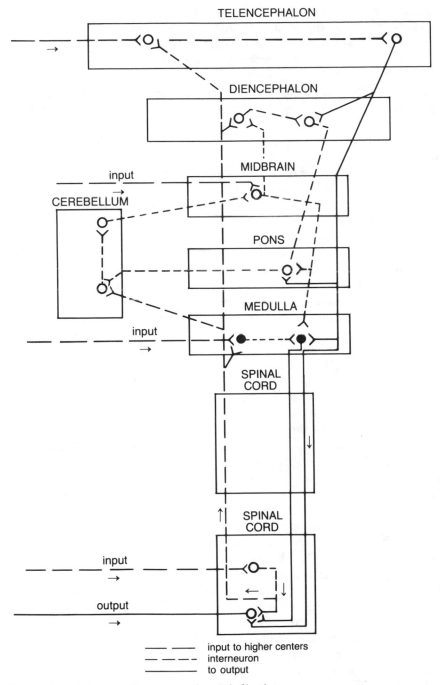

Figure 2.4. Schematic illustration of encephalization.

spinal level include flexor withdrawal, crossed extension, grasp, extensor thrust, Galenté, reflex stepping, automatic extension of the hand, tonic lumbar, and the myotatic stretch reflex (Fiorentino, 1981). A generator control system for movement initiation is also thought to exist at the spinal level (Orlousky, 1972). Although these theories explain how purposeful movement can occur with intact sensory motor systems at the spinal level, flexible, refined, coordinated movement can only occur through the constant interaction and integration of sensory messages from the tactile, proprioceptive, and vestibular afferent network which is achieved at higher levels within the CNS.

Brainstem.   The *medulla, pons,* and *midbrain* are commonly referred to as the brainstem. In these structures are located the afferent and efferent segments from 10 of the 12 cranial nerves and centers for vital functions such as respiration, cardiac control, swallowing, and gag reflexes.

Within the brainstem is an area known as the *reticular system.* Its function is twofold. First, projections from various motor nuclei descend upon the spinal system, facilitating and/or suppressing appropriate motor neurons. This assists in maintaining a readiness-to-fire state within the motor neuronal pool (Granit, 1979). The second function is to awaken or alert the CNS through tracts which ascend upon higher centers. Many CP children have difficulty regulating the reticular system. Excessive activation results in excessive muscle tone and overstimulation of higher centers, resulting in an inability to concentrate, hyperactivity, and even irritability. If the system is suppressed, low muscular tone may result as well as lethargy, a semisleep state, or sluggish responses within higher center processing.

The brainstem structures are not all alike nor do they all provide the same function. In addition to cranial nerve motor function, different areas within this section of the CNS are responsible for specific reflex activity. The tonic labyrinthine, positive supporting, shifting, traction, rooting, and sucking reflexes appear to be processed in the medulla. There is a question about whether the tonic neck reflexes are mediated in the medulla or upper cervical region. Appropriate stimulation to the pons area elicits neck righting, parachute, and pontine posture patterns. Midbrain centers control the body-on-body and body-on-head reflexes, labyrinthine righting, and the Moro reflex (Fiorentino, 1981).

Cerebellum.   The cerebellum functions as the modulator of muscle tone that is essential for posture and movement. This structure receives numerous projections from (a) the spinal system, (b) the brainstem structures, and (c) higher centers. The cerebellum is unable to regulate tone adequately unless the peripheral and higher center system send data to it. Distortion or delays in that incoming data as well as cerebellar lesions can create serious problems in cerebellar output, resulting in deficits in modulation of tone. These deficits create the clinical signs of ataxia.

Diencephalon. Lying between the highest integrative center (cerebral cortex) and the brainstem, the diencephalon functions primarily as a relay network. All sensory stimuli, except olfaction, which reach the cerebral cortex cross synapses within the diencephalon. Because any synaptic junction is a site for diminishing neuronal activity through inhibitory interneurons or heightening activity through facilitory neurons, the diencephalon undoubtedly integrates and refines almost all information going to the cerebral cortex. This integrative center consists of the *thalamus*, the lateral and medial *geniculate bodies*, the *subthalamus*, and the *hypothalamus*.

Not only is the diencephalon a relay center for afferent input originating in the peripheral and cranial nerves going to the cerebral cortex, it is also a vital relay center for information traveling to and from most areas within the CNS. Thus neuronal damage affecting the diencephalon has the potential to indirectly affect functions in almost all areas of the nervous system. For example, a child suffering insult to the medial geniculate body of the thalamus will have difficulty receiving auditory information from cranial nerve VIII. If the lesion is located deep within the associated lobes of the thalamus, communication between sensory processing of auditory input, and motor production of articulated language may be affected or lost. Thus the diencephalon plays a key role in higher level CNS function.

Telencephalon. The telencephalon is the highest and most advanced integrative structure within the human CNS. It consists of three subdivisions—*basal ganglia, limbic lobe*, and *cerebral cortex*—all of which play critical roles in regulating external and internal responses to the world around us. Because their cells need an abundance of oxygen to metabolize and survive, they are surrounded by blood vessels that provide the necessary nutrients. If oxygen is not abundant within the blood supply or the vascular system is damaged, neurological sequelae can be major. Spasticity is associated with lesions in the telencephalon, which is especially susceptible to hypoxic and ischemic insult prior to and at birth.

Basal Ganglia. It is known that the basal ganglia function as a motor generator, but the complexity and specific regulatory function of this intricate neuron structure still baffles basic neuroscientists. The basal ganglia produce both manifestation of tone (a state of preparedness) and postural reflexes, and it is thought to be a major storage center for reflexes categorized as learned. These semiautomatic behaviors include such activities as feeding, dressing, walking, typing, and automatic speech. A lesion or chemical imbalance causing alteration or blockage of function of areas within the basal ganglia will produce signs of proximal rigidity, distal nonintentional tremors, or choreo-athetoid type movement patterns.

Athetosis is a basal ganglia dysfunction resulting from brief, total asphyxia. Usually this insult occurs to a full-term infant suffering a birth trauma. Often these children exhibit hypotonia until approximately 10 to 12 months of age, at which time athetoid CP is confirmed (Ito, 1979). The reason for the delay in presentation of clinical signs can be explained by the myelination patterns within the CNS (Yakovleo & Lecours, 1967). It is not until the latter part of the first year that heavy myelination occurs within the basal ganglia, thus marking the clinical signs.

Limbic Lobe. The limbic lobe is intricately linked with higher and lower centers within the CNS. The limbic system includes many structures other than the limbic lobe. The role of the limbic system is control of olfaction, regulation of visceral responses, emotional responses, memory, and motivation or drive. Obviously many of these roles are critical elements in production of higher order thought processes such as visual-analytical thought and verbal communication. The limbic lobe is surrounded by the lateral and third ventricles; hence, ventricular swelling or vascular problems due to premature birth or trauma at or after birth, can drastically affect the functioning of this system and create symptoms of cerebral palsy.

Cerebral Cortex and Cerebrum. The cerebrum, also called the cortex or neocortex, is the highest integrative center of the CNS. It processes all sensory information projected from lower centers and plans appropriate responses to the events presented in the external environment. The cerebrum is made up of four lobes in each of two hemispheres. Specialization of the hemispheres and the lobes within them allows us to recognize and associate millions of incoming bits of stimuli, put meaning to that information, store it and/or act upon it appropriately. Without this structure we are helpless, yet without the subcortical structures to feed information into the cerebral cortex, the cortex is functionless. The cerebral cortex controls higher order thought leading from interpretation of body image, body schema, sound recognition, and sight recognition to complex intellectual functions of receptive and expressive speech, reading, mathematical computation, graphic art production, complex motor planning, and higher order problem solving. The capacity of the cerebral cortex seems to be infinite. As long as the substructures maintaining the input challenge the cerebral cortex, it seems that the higher structure will try to adapt and learn. For that reason the potential of the CNS to learn is dependent not upon aptitude tests but rather upon the skill of the clinician and/or teacher to provide an appropriate input environment which nurtures higher order thought.

Sensory Systems

Theories of generator control systems and efferent drives at the spinal, cerebellar, and basal ganglia centers have suggested how automatic movement, and even some purposeful movement, can occur without input from sensory systems. However, most purposeful movement is refined, adapted, and coordinated through the integration of exteroceptive (skin), proprioceptive (muscles, joints, tendons), and vestibular messages. The degree of sophistication of fine motor skills required to initiate and carry through a movement pattern is correlated with the CNS ability to receive and integrate sensory messages into meaningful responses. Thus activities such as handwriting or speech production should require a higher degree of sensory integration than gross motor patterns such as walking. This is not to say that CP children cannot talk unless they are able to walk, but it does stress the fact that the fine control over the oral motor system is probably much more complex and dependent on intact sensory reception and integration than that required for a semiautomatic, gross motor activity.

Understanding the neurophysiology of sensory systems is essential in designing therapy to alter motor responses through the use of sensory input. Seven categories of sensory receptors have been generally identified in humans. They are exteroceptive, proprioceptive, vestibular, olfactory, gustatory, auditory, and visual. The separation of input into isolated categories leads to some difficulty due to the interrelationships of various sensory modalities. Some researchers, clinicians, and teachers classify proprioceptive and vestibular input together, referring to the combined sensory messages as kinesthetic input. Separation of vestibular and auditory input into isolated systems negates their relationship at a sensory reception level. Yet prior to understanding the interrelationships of various sensory modalities, identification of the separate characteristics is crucial.

Exteroceptive System (Cutaneous).   The exteroceptive or somatosensory system is usually divided into two distinct systems. The spinothalamic is older and is thought to mediate primitive stimuli for protective responses. The lemniscal has developed more recently and mediates the discriminative aspects of tactile sensitivity. The two systems have distinct anatomical and physiological characteristics.

Lemniscal System.   The lemniscal system has clearly defined pathways. Orderly spatial topographic representation of the surface of the skin within this tract system enables the CNS to discriminate specific tactile stimuli. Proprioceptive input is also transmitted through this system. With tactile and proprioceptive stimuli ascending together, information about touch, pressure, contour, quality, localization, and spatial details of mechanical stimuli can be processed by the parietal lobes and discriminatory meaning given to that information. This tract system plays a key role in fine motor integration or the lack thereof, if a deficit is present as in CP.

Spinothalamic System.   The spinothalamic tract is not well defined neuroanatomically. It elicits reflex activity at the spinal level. Flexor withdrawal is an example of the motor response pattern to a tactile stimulus such as a pinprick. Nondiscriminatory cutaneous input via the trigeminal nerve entering the CNS at the medulla can also elicit withdrawal type patterns within the mouth or facial region. In addition to influence over spinal and brainstem reflex loops, the afferents within the spinothalamic tracts, as well as those projecting from the spinal cord itself, send large numbers of collateral projections into the reticular activating system in the brainstem.

Due to the interrelationship of the spinothalamic system, the reticular formation, and the autonomic nervous system (ANS), the nondiscriminatory exteroceptive system plays a key role in arousing the CNS to potentially harmful stimuli. Perception of pain, light touch, aversive stimuli, protective responses, and pleasurable sexual sensations are functions related to this system.

Some researchers (Poggio & Mountcastle, 1960) suggest that the lemniscal system has an inhibitory influence over the spinothalamic system. As an individual develops more highly differentiated touch, protective responses diminish and are only elicited when needed. For example, a young child tends to withdraw from any touch stimuli. As the child matures and the lemniscal system myelinates, the child learns to discriminate between touch and harmful touch such as a tack or a hot stove. Ayers (1980) has postulated that a child who shows a hypersensitivity to touch (touch or tactile defensiveness) may have an overreactive spinothalamic system and an underdeveloped lemniscal system. Hyperactive tongue thrust which prevents good feeding and oral motor control would be another example of the imbalance in these two exteroceptive systems.

Treatment alternatives that focus upon the receptor sensitivity of the exteroceptive system are varied and numerous, yet general characteristics can be identified. Any stimulus—whether it be cold, touch, or pain—that elicits a full or partial phasic withdrawal will tend to increase the CNS excitatory level as well as cause specific motor responses. Any stimulus that is sustained—such as cold, neutral (i.e., body temperature) warmth, maintained pressure, or slow continuous stroking—will tend to facilitate the adaptation of many cutaneous receptors, thus decreasing input, decreasing reticular activity, and often decreasing muscle excitation underlying the stimulated skin.

Proprioceptive System.   The proprioceptive system includes all sensory receptors originating in the muscles, tendons, and joints.

Muscle.   Sensory receptors responsive to stretch are found in muscles within a smaller structure, the muscle spindle. These receptors inform the spinal system, the cerebellum, and the cerebral cortex of the degree and type of stretch placed on every muscle within the body. Stretch receptors are activated by external factors such as gravity.

The internal environment, controlled and modified by the CNS, also affects the spindle through the use of a small motor neuron (gamma) which causes intrafusal muscle fibers within the spindle to contract. This activates the sensory receptors through stretch (internal stretch). Both internal and external stretch (produced by gravity, positioning, and therapeutic procedures) regulate the muscle spindle afferent responses. The intricate balance of internal and external stretch is a key element in coordinating movement. If there is too little internal stretch (hypotonia) then the muscle cannot respond appropriately to the demands of the external environment. If, on the other hand, the internal stretch is excessive (spasticity), the muscle stretch overreacts to slight external stretch which also prevents the muscle from responding appropriately. Some forms of cerebral palsy drastically alter the ongoing stretch sensitivity of the spindle afferents via efferent activity. This, in turn, drastically alters their ability to respond to and control the demands placed upon them by their external environment.

Because the spindle afferents are stretch receptors, any treatment procedure which utilizes stretch as its input will affect this system. Techniques of quick stretch, tapping, resistance, vibration, positioning, electrical stimulation, active motion, and many others all fall into the same sensory categorization schema. The ultimate goal of any of these procedures is to facilitate higher center control over the gamma motor neuron and thus the spindle afferent's sensitivity to stretch.

Tendon Organs. Muscles are attached to bones by tendons, within which tension receptors called tendon organs (TO) are located. Tendon organs respond to active muscle contraction (Houk & Henneman, 1967) and they respond throughout the normal range of active motion (Rymer, Houk, & Crago, 1979).

The role of the tendon organ is twofold. First, at the spinal level or, in the case of facial muscles, lower medulla level, it inhibits the muscle attached to the tendon and facilitates the antagonist. This physiological relationship is utilized in many therapeutic procedures in order to modify hyperactive or spastic muscles. For example, if extreme stretch is used on spastic muscles, inhibition via TO can occur and will be maintained as long as the stretch is continued. Simultaneously, facilitation of what is usually a hypotonic antagonist is also being recruited via the TO. The second and primary function of the TO is to inform higher centers, especially the cerebellum, regarding the degree of tension being exerted on the tendon. In this way the cerebellum can regulate the degree of neuroexcitation placed on motor neurons and thus better adapt to external demands.

Joints. Joint receptors are found in articulating surfaces between two or more bones. There are four major types of joint receptors (Wyke, 1972). Type I joint receptors are stimulated by both static and dynamic joint tension or muscle pull, and the response generated is thought to be postural hold and position sense. Clinically, by adding heavy joint approximation or tension, better postural holding patterns should develop. By taking away that approximation, holding patterns should decrease and movement should develop. These techniques are often used to facilitate neck, trunk, shoulder, and hip postural control.

Type II receptors are stimulated by dynamic or sudden changes in joint tension. It is hypothesized that the CNS uses input from these receptors to develop awareness of joint motion and range. The combined input of Type I and II joint receptors helps us control our movement in space and provides the basis for developing certain movement-related abilities.

Type III receptors are stimulated by sudden or dynamic changes within the joints at the extreme ranges of movement and help to prevent hyperextension of the joint.

Type IV receptors are stimulated by pain. Their function is protective; they inhibit muscle contraction to avoid further joint damage.

Vestibular System.   The vestibular apparatus is proprioceptive in function and is often combined with the body proprioceptors to form the kinesthetic system. Functionally, the vestibular system is responsible for static horizontal positioning, dynamic maintenance of the head in a face-vertical position, and head and body equilibrium responses. Yet the vestibular system seldom works in isolation from other sensory systems. In conjunction with the tactile and proprioceptive systems, it drastically affects muscle tone both during postural holding and movement. The vestibular system's interrelationship with vision leads to function of visual gaze, head-eye directed movement, and directionality. The vestibular system's impact on attention, learning, and emotional development cannot be ignored (Wilson & Peterson, 1980).

Anatomically, the vestibular system consists of a vestibule and three semicircular canals in each ear. The vestibule, which is referred to as the static labyrinth, elicits tonic reflexes in response to static and dynamic changes in position and to gravitational influences. The three semicircular canals respond to angular or rotatory acceleration or deceleration of the head. Their role, unlike the vestibule, is control of ocular movement, equilibrium, and active movement.

Because the vestibular apparatus has such diffuse connections, it is a unique sensory modality. It has the capacity to cause tremendous facilitory and inhibitory influences over muscle tone; ANS regulation; reticular and limbic activity influencing attention, memory, and motivation; as well as higher order learning within the various lobes of the cerebral cortex. Techniques which alter the state of neuroexcitation of the vestibular system are divided into two groups: facilitory or inhibitory. Techniques which slow the firing of either the vestibule or semicircular canal receptors tend to suppress the influence of the vestibular system. Procedures which facilitate the receptors will heighten the vestibular responses. For example, slow rocking of a hyperactive and/or extremely spastic child may decrease exaggerated responses, while fast rocking may heighten them (Umphred & McCormach, 1985).

Olfactory System. How receptor cells located in the roof of the nasal cavity transduce odors into meaningful perceptions is not well understood, but it appears to be a chemical process (Afifi & Bergman, 1980). From these odor-sensitive receptors, impulses are transmitted directly to the temporal lobe. Unlike all other sensory systems, the impulses do not pass through or synapse in the thalamus (Cain, 1974). Olfactory projections from the temporal lobes are thought to influence behavior and emotions. Noxious or unpleasant odors can facilitate protective responses such as withdrawal, sneezing, and choking. Sharp smells such as ammonia can heighten alertness of the CNS but also may cause reflex interruption of breathing. Pleasant odors can evoke strong mood changes and heighten the senses.

This potential for alteration of CNS responses has led to the use of odors in therapeutic procedures. Because there has been little research in the area, therapists should exercise caution in using this modality. Some children, especially those with head trauma or inflammatory disorders, seem to be hypersensitive to smells. Therapists and teachers must be aware of the external olfactory environment surrounding the child, especially if the child is experiencing dramatic mood changes without any apparent cause.

Gustatory System. Taste involves a chemical process which is derived not only from food but also from smell, temperature, and texture. The primary taste senses (salty, sweet, bitter, and sour) combine to create a larger number of perceived tastes. Areas of the tongue vary in sensitivity to the four primary tastes. The tip of the tongue detects sweet, the base detects bitter, and the sides are particularly sensitive to sour.

Because gustatory sensation is generally used in feeding and prefeeding activities, the complexity of this sense needs to be understood. The oral region is sensitive to pressure, texture, and temperature as well as taste; for that reason, sensory input such as mashed bananas versus mashed apples may create varied responses in the child. Both are sweet, but the textures differ greatly. A therapist needs to be aware of the emotional responses of a child during feeding in order to obtain maximum responses. The reader is referred to Chapter 7 on Prespeech and Feeding Development for additional information.

Visual System. The eye is the most complex of the sensory receptors. For a review of the anatomy of the eye and the processing of visual information, refer to Chapter 6, Visual Problems.

Because the visual system is so complex, it is often used by physicians for diagnosing CNS disorders. Similarly, the visual system can be used as an input modality for a large variety of treatment procedures. These procedures can vary from simple input changes such as hues, lighting, colors, to complex procedures such as those described in Chapter 6. The clinician must remember that any visual input is a potential treatment procedure. Thus a change in lighting (either type or intensity) or color (red versus blue mat) may alter the child's responses during treatment.

Familiarity with the visual-perceptual system and its interrelationship to all therapeutic settings is crucial if an optimal environment for learning is to be created. Consider the visual input and complexity of the visual array if, for example, during a speech session the child is facing the therapist and behind the therapist is (a) a blank wall, (b) a window, or (c) a large therapy room full of people. Whether the child's visual processing is intact or deficient, the therapy session will be distinctly different in each of these situations.

Auditory System. The anatomy and physiology of the hearing mechanism are described in Chapter 5. The complexity of this system leads to the use of audition in numerous treatment modalities. Once auditory input enters the CNS, its pathways become diffuse (Williams & Warwick, 1975).

Some collaterals project to the reticular activating system through which sound stimuli alert the CNS. Others go to the cerebellum and enable the body to respond quickly with a motor action in the event of a sudden, loud, or unfamiliar noise. It is important for therapists to bear in mind that auditory input might have either a facilitory or inhibitory influence on CNS activity. The quality and intensity of the therapist's or teacher's voice may drastically alter reticular level activity and thus influence attention, memory, learning, and motor response. The speaker's affective state as revealed by the voice can have an effect on the child's responses. Extraneous noise which teachers and therapists ignore may be disturbing to the child.

Combined Sensory Input. Although the mode of entry of a specific therapeutic procedure may focus upon one sensory system, all techniques have the potential of being multisensory. For example, proprioceptive facilitation requires that the skin be touched, thus stimulating tactile receptors. Tactile stimulation may facilitate autonomic receptors. Many techniques intentionally employ multiple modalities in order to gain optimal facilitation.

The importance of understanding the neuromechanism cannot be overstressed. Random facilitation through cross-modality stimulation can prevent learning as easily as it can enhance development. For that reason many therapists use only one approach to treatment such as sensory integration (SI), neurodevelopmental therapy (NDT), or behavioral modification. When comprehensive understanding of an approach is lacking but knowledge of the sequences and application methods unique to that technique are known, a therapist often feels obligated to implement procedures inherent only to that method. On the other hand, a clinician who understands why something is or is not effective, and understands the options available to create alternative treatment methods to facilitate the same response, has the flexibility to learn any method while being receptive to alternative ideas (Umphred & McCormach, 1985).

Motor Systems

There are two primary motor systems. One controls movement, the other posture. The two systems work together in an intricate way to regulate specific motor output. The end result of each system's functioning is muscle contraction. Therapists evaluate CNS functioning through observation of this contraction or lack thereof when, for example, the child is asked (or shown how) to swallow, roll over, or say "ah." To make appropriate motor responses to specific input, a complex interaction of sensory processing associations, motor planning, and motor responses must be integrated. If the child fails at the task, questions arise regarding which system (from input to output) is causing the dysfunction. Because children with CP characteristically have poor control over motor responses, it is essential that therapists understand how motor output is controlled.

Muscle contraction is controlled by motor neurons whose firing patterns are regulated by interneurons originating from various levels within the CNS. The firing patterns regulating movement are different from those controlling posture. The postural system elicits *simultaneous* firing of agonistic and antagonistic muscles surrounding joints, especially proximal ones. The movement systems employ a *reciprocal* firing pattern causing the agonist to contract as the antagonist relaxes. With the postural system causing muscles around the joint to contract simultaneously, while the movement system facilitates other muscles to produce motion, an interaction develops which allows unlimited variation in the force, speed, direction, and thus control over the movement pattern.

Movement. There seem to be movement generators at various levels within the CNS (Jewell, 1985; Orlousky, 1972). A generator at the spinal level facilitates extension, and another reciprocally elicits flexion. These generators are triggered both by peripheral afferents such as light touch, or by extrasegmental interneurons within the cord or from higher centers. Many types of sensory input through interneuronal connections influence these motor generators. The neck proprioceptors which elicit the tonic neck reflexes, or the labyrinthine neurons producing the tonic labyrinthine reflexes, are just a few. Touch or texture to the tongue producing a thrust pattern would be another example.

Control and modification of these basic movement generators have evolved with the development of the cerebellum, diencephalon, and telencephalon. As the afferent system became more specialized, processing of sensory input became more complex and refined, leading to higher regulation over the movement system. Regulation comes not only at the beginning of a motor plan. By using continuous feedback from afferent neurons, movement is modified and refined throughout the activity.

The cerebellum plays a key role in generating tone. It affects the rate, direction, distance, and strength of a movement but does not seem to create new programs. A child with only a cerebellar lesion will thus have the ability to modify the spinal and brainstem movement generators through higher center control, but will have difficulty controlling the rate, direction, range, and reciprocal muscle interaction during the movement pattern. This problem is seen in congenital and traumatic cerebellar insults in ataxic CP children.

Program generators within the basal ganglia produce both ballistic and slow movements (Jewell, 1985). A subthalamic nucleus lesion produces the disturbed ballistic movements seen in children with choreoathetosis. Nonintentional tremor seen in some CP children, especially in the distal aspect of the tongue, is probably a pattern that originates in the basal ganglia.

Both the prefrontal and frontal lobe areas of the cerebral cortex are processing and control centers for movement. Once a sensory-motor plan is formulated by the sensory processing systems, that information is sent to the frontal lobes which then send motor commands to the basal ganglia, cerebellum, brainstem, and spinal areas to regulate this goal-directed activity through the modification of all the movement generators. The cerebral cortex coordinates the slow and fast movements mediated by the basal ganglia, the regulation of tone by the cerebellum, and the phasic and tonic reflex activity of the brainstem and spinal system in order to orchestrate the entire sequence of motor events with refinement and total control.

The CNS modifies movement not only by facilitating or inhibiting the movement generators. It controls and modifies movement by regulating the degree of postural tone released to stabilize the joint structures, thus slowing or stopping the movement.

Posture. Posture is often equated with static, rigid, or tonic muscle contraction. Normal postures, however, are extremely dynamic and vary with the slightest alteration in body alignment. They change from limb to limb, segment to segment, or total body to position in space. The postural system not only allows a person to remain vertical by constantly readjusting the posture as the body sways over its base of support, it also controls and modifies movement by slowing down the rate of contraction or by stopping a contraction at the end of the range to avoid subluxation.

Development and constant integration of the postural system relies on input from the proprioceptive and vestibular systems. Normally vision also plays a key role in facilitating "uprightness" against gravity; however, vision can be lost without loss of postural control. The muscles most involved in posture are proximally located antigravity muscles. The background neural activity necessary for postural control seems to be present at the spinal and brainstem level, but the control over that neuroexcitation is thought to be regulated at a much higher level—possibly the basal ganglia because of its unique influence over postural holding.

Postural control regulates both extensor and flexor activity simultaneously. If too much tone is generated, the postural system modifies it; this is true of either flexor or extensor tone. A large amount of antigravity extensor tone is generated in the lower brainstem, while flexor tone is generated in the midbrain. A lesion in the basal ganglia, limbic system, or cortical structures may cause the child to lose the ability to regulate the generated tone. Muscle tone without higher center control produces the clinical sign of spasticity. Spasticity is not too much postural tone but rather too much tone, which may affect only one side of the joint or may be symmetrical around the joint.

Disturbances in posture can vary from low postural tone, as seen in the athetoid child, to too much tone as seen in the spastic diplegic and quadraplegic. Low tone can be caused by many problems—afferent damage, or cerebellar and central brainstem lesions. Increasing that tone becomes a primary clinical goal, no matter the disability or the treatment approach implemented. The proprioceptive, vestibular, and visual input systems are primary modalities for postural integration; thus using these systems to create tone would be a method of choice. Not only should muscle tone be produced, but control over that tone is necessary if postural regulation is to be achieved; hence, the child needs to experience the holding of a posture as well as have opportunities to control and modify this increased tone while engaged in purposeful activity.

Although low postural tone can be seen in some CP children, too much tone is much more commonly observed. This tone is often present in antigravity extensors due to the reflexes originating in spinal and brainstem nuclei. Regulation of this tone is a key to postural development. If an antigravity muscle is spastic (increase in stretch sensitivity), then lowering neuroexcitation on the motor neurons innervating that muscle is important. Several methods can be used to directly or indirectly cause such a change in interneuronal firing. The end result is not to stop contraction of the spastic muscle, but rather to regulate and control its firing and the firing pattern of its antagonist.

Higher Center Control

Posture and movement systems must be controlled together in order to manufacture the specific patterns of neuroexcitation required for any and all goal-directed movement. The finer the movement, the more integrated that control must become. Speech is an excellent example of this intricate interaction of posture and movement. Posture of the neck and the back of the tongue lead to control over the placement of the distal aspect of the tongue during speech. The postural interaction of the trunk extensors and abdominal flexors, along with the reciprocal movement patterns of muscles of respiration, lead to controlled exhalation required for speech production. No matter the inherent cognitive potential of a CP child, without the posture and movement base leading to trunk, neck, and oral motor control, production of intelligible speech is virtually impossible.

The cerebral cortex seems to be the location that ultimately regulates the motor system, thus controlling movement and posture. Higher center processing of sensory input and relaying that data to motor areas is an important element in regulation of motor output. Apraxia results when higher center processing or relaying of sensory data is impaired. Deficits produced by higher center lesions can be devastating to any child, but especially to a child who also has a lesion in lower order motor systems.

The emotional or limbic system has a potent influence over the motor systems and generation of tone. Most adults are aware when they are "uptight" or under a lot of pressure due to their neuromuscular responses. When upset, an intact CNS creates tone by activating the reticular system, thus indirectly eliciting alpha motor neuron firing. A CP child is no different. When that child is upset, an increase in tone or lack of control over the generated tone will occur naturally. When the child is calm and relaxed, less emotional tone will be produced and better control observed. The limbic system is also involved in attention and memory which are essential to learning. A child who is placed in painful physical or emotional surroundings will not show the same rate of learning as a child with identical deficits who is placed in an enriched learning environment. Similarly, a child should not be expected to perform a fine motor task such as speaking when positioned in a pattern which requires a high degree of cortical control. Even children who are cognitively capable of higher order tasks such as speaking or reading, may fail to acquire these skills if they have to use too much energy and attention to control a sitting position. Failure creates pain and frustration which heighten emotional tone, making it harder to succeed at the task.

HIGHER ORDER PROCESSING AND LEARNING

Many of the topics discussed in this book involve methods of stimulating higher order processing and learning in order to achieve a desired response. Any time a behavioral response is elicited through specific input, higher processing systems have been activated. The major obstacle to learning in CP children may not be their CNS malfunction but our failure to create the correct environment and provide appropriate learning experiences for them.

An outstanding feature of higher order processing centers is hemispheric specialization. This might be viewed as a division of labor of interneurons within the various cortical regions; however, this division does not seem to be static. Information is transmitted to both sides of the brain, but each hemisphere processes the afferent inputs differently and for different content. In most humans, the right hemisphere analyzes the content for its spatial or global characteristics. This content can be auditory, visual, proprioceptive, tactile, vestibular, or any other modality. The left hemisphere analyzes content for its temporal sequencing or the step-by-step sequence of the event. The right temporal lobe processes tone and rhythm of voice, while the left is involved in the production of and sequencing of sound. The right frontal lobe is responsible for the whole body's action in motor planning or body-in-space types of tasks, while the left frontal lobe sequences the motor acts or motor planning. Certain cognitive strategies such as speech or reading tend to have a strong temporal component, while math tends to be more spatial. Yet both sides of the brain are important in all higher cognitive processing.

From this review of the neurophysiologic bases of current treatment procedures, it is apparent that no area of the CNS functions in isolation. There is interdependence between lower and higher structures and within structures at the same level. It appears that all systems have the ability to exert influence over all other systems. This makes it plausible that behavioral output may be modified and sequenced through a variety of input methods.

CONCLUSION

Current approaches to the treatment of cerebral palsy base their rationale and procedures on interpretation of CNS functioning; however, our understanding of the brain and its intricate neuromechanisms is yet at an elementary level. The rationale for any approach is open to challenge and may prove to be wrong. Yet the normal behaviors, improved quality of life, and higher degree of independence achieved through current approaches cannot be denied. Even though clinical experience demonstrates the efficacy of any method, the underlying rationale may need upgrading as brain research improves.

The four approaches used most frequently in clinical and academic settings are neurodevelopmental therapy (NDT), sensory integrative therapy (SI), behavioral modification, and cognitive training or retraining. Each one of these methods has the potential to help some neurologically handicapped children. Yet the methods differ in their major focus on CNS processing. Any one child may show little or no improvement if the approach employed does not match the level of his or her CNS integration. Effective treatment requires an understanding of the neurophysiologic and neuropsychologic principles on which the technique is based and comprehension of how the child receives, processes, and responds to stimulation.

Neurodevelopmental Therapy (NDT)

NDT rationale is based on the assumption that children need to experience and learn normal automatic movement before they can volitionally carry out an activity. Facilitation of normal righting reactions emphasizing rotation (brainstem), postural control (basal ganglia), and equilibrium reactions (cerebral cortex) is a key to unlocking normal movement. The rotatory component of all movement patterns is stressed. It is theorized that once these reactions have been facilitated through handling the child in various spatial and developmental positions, the child should automatically take control. At that time the child would demonstrate higher level motor control and thus a more highly integrated CNS. Although facilitation is elicited through sensory input and perceptual and cognitive processing of that data, the focus is not on perception and cognition but rather on motor control. Thus NDT is especially appropriate for young CP children or children with poor motor control (Campbell, 1984).

Sensory Integrative Therapy (SI)

SI emphasizes the child's active participation in the learning environment and the child's need to integrate multisensory input in order to achieve higher perceptual-cognitive learning. Although the focus, as in NDT, is on identification of a child's developmental delays and lack of neurologic integration, the major population receiving therapy is learning disabled children (LD). In this group, the delays or gaps treated reflect CNS development associated with cognitive-perceptual functioning at a two- to four-year developmental level. The brainstem and basal ganglia problems focused upon in NDT are not usually the primary deficits of the children receiving SI therapy. These children reflect problems in the reticular-limbic systems, the cortical receiving and association areas leading to deficits in motor output. Treating the attention, bilateral integration, praxis, spatial processing, and other perceptual problems assists the child in further integrating his or her CNS and improving overall performance (Ayers, 1980).

Behavior Modification

A behavior modification approach assumes that behavior can be changed through successive positive reinforcement toward a desired goal. This approach is most effective with children who have minimal motor involvement and limited cognitive abilities. It does not require a high level of cognitive processing (cortex) by the child but does require the integration of a large number of lower centers within the CNS. The therapist using this method tries to elicit more normal, socially acceptable, or functional responses by the child. For example, if the child has the motor potential to be a self-feeder but does not understand at a cognitive level what is required, the task can be broken into small steps. As the child approximates success within each step, strong positive feedback is given. As each step is mastered, the next is begun until the child has succeeded at the entire activity. At that time the behavior is semiautomatic. This approach uses the limbic system's influences over motivation, and the control of the basal ganglia and lower CNS centers over semiautomatic responses. Although this method can be extremely effective for some children, a CP child with severe motor problems does not always have the potential to learn movement through reinforcement alone. A child with an asymmetrical tonic neck reflex which straightens the arm when the face is directed toward that extremity would never be able to bring the hand to mouth if behavior modification techniques alone were used. When the same child throws a temper tantrum, however, this approach could succeed because the child has the ability to change that specific behavior (Craighead, Kazdin, & Mahoney, 1981).

Cognitive Training

Cognitive training or retraining has developed out of an education model and focuses on cortical function and ability to learn if the learning environment is appropriate to the child's level of processing. Assessment of the child's cognitive abilities allows the therapist or educator to identify intact cognitive processes as well as deficit systems. The cognitive systems which are intact are used as primary strategies to achieve attention and learning in all facets of education. The deficit systems are not ignored but remediated through sequential treatment strategies designed to improve the deficient cognitive skills. It is assumed that since the cortex controls all areas of the CNS, it can be used to control any deficit system. This approach has proved successful with cognitive processing and memory deficits but, as with all approaches, not all children respond optimally. Many of our response patterns use automatic or semiautomatic motor plans. The higher cortical system should elicit these automatic plans rather than plan each component of a child's movement. If cognitive training is used to teach a child to move or to hold a position such as sitting, then tremendous cortical control will be used for this task, thus limiting the cortical energy available for higher thought (Ben-Yishay & Diller, 1981).

Each of the procedures described, as well as all other approaches, has strengths and weaknesses. Some techniques will work with some children, some with others, but no one approach works optimally on all children or for all professionals. Clinicians and teachers can increase their clinical and academic expertise through learning about brain function.

REFERENCES

Afifi, A., & Bergman, R. (1980). *Basic neuroscience.* Baltimore: Urban and Schwarzenbert.

Ayers, A. J. (1980). *Sensory integration and the child.* Los Angeles: Western Psychological Services.

Ben-Yishay, Y., & Diller, L. (1981). Cognitive remediation. In M. Rosenthal, E. R. Griffith, M. R. Bond, & J. D. Miller (Eds.), *Rehabilitation of head injured adults* (pp. 367–380). Philadelphia: F. A. Davis.

Cain, W. S. (Ed.). (1974). Odors, evaluation utilization and control. *Annual NY Academy Science,* 2371–2439.

Campbell, S. (Ed.). (1984). *Pediatric neurological disorders.* New York: Churchill Livingstone.

Coleman, M. (1981). Congenital brain syndromes. In M. Coleman (Ed.), *Neonatal neurology* (pp. 371–384). Baltimore: University Park Press.

Craighead, W. E., Kazdin, A. E., & Mahoney, M. J. (1981). *Behavioral modification.* Boston: Houghton Mifflin.

Fiorentino, M. A. (1981). *A basis for sensorimotor development: Normals/abnormal.* Springfield, IL: Charles C Thomas.

Granit, R. R. (1979). Interpretation of supraspinal effects on the gamma system. In R. Granit (Ed.), *Progress in brain research, 50*(147) (pp. 147–154). Netherlands: North Hollands Biomedical Press.

Held, R. (1965). Plasticity in sensory-motor systems. *Scientific America, 213,* 84–94.

Houk, J. C., & Henneman, E. (1967). Responses of golgi tendon organs to active contractions of the soleus muscle of the cat. *Journal of Neurophysiology, 30,* 466–481.

Illingsworth, R. S. (1980). *The development of the infant and young child: Abnormal and normal* (7th ed.). Edinburgh: Churchill Livingstone.

Ito, M. (1979). Computed tomography of cerebral palsy: Evaluation of brain damage by volume index of CSF space. *Brain Development, 4,* 293.

Jewell, M. J. (1985). Neuroanatomical correlation of reflexes, reactions and behaviors with levels of central nervous system organization. In D. A. Umphred (Ed.), *Neurological rehabilitation* (pp. 26–40). St. Louis: C. V. Mosby.

Orlousky, G. N. (1972). The effect of different descending systems on flexor and extensor activity during locomotion. *Brain Research, 40,* 359.

Page, K. E., & Wigglesworth, J. S. (1979). Haemorrhage, ischemis, and the perinatal brain, *Clinics in developmental medicine, 69 & 70.* Philadelphia: Lippincott.

Poggio, G. F., & Mountcastle, V. B. (1960). A study of the functional contribution of the lemniscal and spinothalamic systems to somatic sensibility. *Bulletin John Hopkins Hospital, 106,* 266–316.

Pribram, K. H. (1971). *Language of the brain: Experimental paradoxes and principles in neurophysiology.* Englewood Cliffs, NJ: Prentice Hall.

Rymer, W. Z., Houk, J. C., & Crago, P. E. (1979). Mechanisms of the clasp-knife reflex studied in an animal model. *Experimental Brain Research, 37,* 93–113.

Umphred, D. A., & McCormach, G. (1985). Classification of common facilitory and inhibitory treatment techniques. In D. A. Umphred (Ed.), *Neurological rehabilitation* (pp. 72–117). St. Louis: C. V. Mosby.

Vining, E. (1976). Cerebral palsy: A pediatric developmentalist's overview. *American Journal of Disabled Children, 130,* 643–649.

Volpe, J. J. (1981). *Neurology of the newborn.* Philadelphia: W. B. Saunders.

Volpe, J. J., & Koenigsberger, R. (1981). Neurologic disorders. In G. B. Avery (Ed.), *Neonatology* (2nd ed.) (pp. 910–963). Philadelphia: Lippincott.

Williams, P. L., & Warwick, R. (1975). *Functional neuroanatomy of man.* Philadelphia: W. B. Saunders.

Wilson, V., & Peterson, B. (1980). The role of the vestibular system in posture and movement. In V. B. Mountcastle, *Medical physiology* (Vol. 2, 14th ed.) (pp. 813–836). St. Louis: C. V. Mosby.

Wyke, B. (1972). Articular neurology—a review. *Physiotherapy, 23,* 94.

Yakovleo, P. I., & Lecours, A. R. (1967). The mylogenetic cycles of regional maturation of the brain. In A. Hinkowski (Ed.), *Regional development of the brain in early life.* (pp. 3–71). Oxford: Blackwell Scientific.

CHAPTER 3

Intellectual Development and Assessment

Joseph L. French

While acknowledging that it is often difficult to assess the psychoeducational status of children with cerebral palsy, French asserts that valid assessment is both possible and essential. Of the many factors reviewed in a comprehensive assessment, level of intellectual functioning is probably most important in determining how children learn. Many instruments and techniques are available for assessment, but knowledge about cerebral palsy and supervised experience with cerebral palsied persons is essential to using them appropriately.

1. *How does French distinguish between* testing *and* assessment *and why is this distinction important?*
2. *What nonintellectual factors affect how people use their intellectual ability, and how might these nonintellectual factors work adversely in cerebral palsy?*
3. *What can be done to maximize a child's performance on a test?*
4. *List examples of test items or types of tests that correlate highly with school achievement but are inappropriate for children with cerebral palsy.*
5. *How do intelligence tests differ from achievement tests? Why is information from both types of tests needed in educational planning for a cerebral palsied child?*

INTRODUCTION

It is difficult to assess the psychoeducational status of children with cerebral palsy, especially those with poor communication skills and poor arm and hand control. The more associated problems present, the more difficult the psychologist's task. Yet, valid assessment is possible and essential. Unfortunately, during their training, most psychologists have not had an opportunity to work with a cerebral palsied child and, as a result, are unable, as practicing psychologists, to make appropriate assessments of the cognitive ability and especially the intellectual capability of physically disabled clients. Reports from psychologists unaccustomed to working with the physically disabled are seldom consistent. Some psychologists, overwhelmed by a child's inability to use traditional patterns of speech and/or to manipulate objects quickly, underestimate—sometimes grossly—the ability of the child to think purposefully. Others, failing to observe the manipulative behaviors of a hopeful mother, overestimate the capability of the child. Some mildly physically handicapped children assumed to be physically average—or nearly so—are incorrectly penalized by examiners choosing tests which include such things as speed of response, correctness of physical movements, and/or correctness of speech in the process of sampling intellectual behavior.

To determine a cerebral palsied child's level of cognitive functioning requires sufficient knowledge about (a) cerebral palsy, (b) the foundations of the assessment process, and (c) appropriate instruments and techniques. Then, with that knowledge, a psychologist needs *many* experiences in working with cerebral palsied individuals under the supervision of a mentor with both this knowledge and considerable experience with such children.

This book provides information about many aspects of cerebral palsy, but an understanding of the condition can be gained only through working with persons who have cerebral palsy. Similarly, this chapter provides an introduction to testing and assessment but does not substitute for a graduate level course in this area, including supervised experience in assessment of persons handicapped by cerebral palsy.

THE ASSESSMENT PROCESS

Testing is often used as a synonym for *assessment*, but the terms are not synonymous. Distinguishing between the two is especially important when developing programs for persons with cerebral palsy. Selection of appropriate educational methods and materials, therapeutic procedures, vocational goals, and living arrangements requires extensive information about the capabilities, limitations, and other characteristics of the client. Comprehensive knowledge cannot be obtained through testing alone. A broader approach to assessment is required.

Contribution of Testing

Testing is often a basic and important ingredient in assessment. A test is a psychoeducational tool which yields a score. A group test provides only a score. A short, individually administered test which takes only a few minutes' time provides little more than a score. Longer, individually administered tests allow the psychologist, within the structure of the testing situation, to probe and to modify procedures to bring out the best of a person. They also provide the psychologist with the opportunity to observe such attitudinal variables as persistence, enthusiasm for the tasks, and consideration of options before making a decision. By adapting procedures for the individual, more accurate scores are obtained. By observing the test-taking behavior of the individual, the psychologist can provide, in addition to the score, a professional evaluation of an initial assessment of the client in that situation. Such observations include perceptions which are difficult to quantify, and for which reliability estimation is difficult.

Tests yield scores for which reliability and validity can be estimated. Tests which have been standardized on a representative sample of a specified population provide specific meaning about what is known, and how much learning has been accomplished. Many of the tests described in the Appendix have been developed and standardized so that comparisons can be made with individuals throughout the mainland U.S. When evaluating performance of children, it is important to know both what the child can do and how others of similar age and experience perform on the same tasks in order to put the information into perspective. When conclusions based on test scores obtained by the psychologist, as a result of a behavior sample collected alone with the child, vary markedly from the psychologist's observations of the child in other situations or from the observations of another professional, additional evidence needs to be collected that is relevant to the question(s) which caused the referral to be made.

Contribution of Assessment

The process of assessment implies the use of comprehensive and complex procedures. Assessment includes interpretation of information from tests and other sources such as rating scales, interviews, and systematic observations; and involves evaluation, interpretation, and appraisal of performance. Assessment should include a variety of behavior samples obtained in each of several settings. Observations in some settings should be repeated frequently enough to obtain satisfactory reliability. All of this information should result in, among other things, an analysis of the characteristics which will predict the child's educability in various settings.

Information obtained in the assessment process should include the child's behavior in school settings and in social systems outside of the class. Observation and measurement of a child's ability while in a testing room with a psychologist may develop one picture of the child's abilities and needs; but observation of a child in the classroom, in the home, or with peers in non-school, non-home conditions may yield different pictures of that child's abilities and needs. Many observations are factual and correct: "Bobby always tells us when he needs to eliminate." "Jane can read and enjoy the humor in the Peanuts comic strip." "Jimmy can match the four basic colors." Other information is not so easily evaluated: "Nancy catches on rapidly and easily." "Although Peter can't speak, he knows everything I say." "Joe could solve that problem if he would."

Information provided by personnel in other disciplines (e.g., teachers, educational specialists, and therapists) about such items as what the child has learned and how many repetitions were necessary may significantly alter the psychologist's interpretation of a test score. Therefore, an evaluation by one person in one situation may be enhanced by observations based on different instruments and/or techniques and by other professionals. An assessment by one professional is more than the sum of the test scores, since it involves an integration of all of the data that are relevant to the situation. An assessment by a multidisciplinary team is more comprehensive than an assessment by one of its members, since it is more extensive in terms of the information available. The quality of a multidisciplinary assessment, as with all assessments, depends upon the quality of the information received and the perceptions of the team members as they render professional judgments.

A comprehensive assessment is never complete. There is always more information to obtain, to integrate, and to judge. Evaluation of information collected about a client by a psychologist about one attribute (e.g., scholastic aptitude) at one time may differ from an evaluation by the same psychologist of the same person in a different social and/or cultural situation. Also, observing the client responding to different tests and different procedures or processes may provide information which modifies the initial assessment.

THE MEASUREMENT OF INTELLIGENCE

Among the many factors which affect how children learn, their level of intellectual functioning is probably the most important. Many parents—and some professional workers—doubt that it is possible to determine the intellectual level of a child with cerebral palsy. While difficult, valid estimates can be made by properly trained and experienced psychologists.

The term IQ is not a synonym for intelligence. IQ, or intelligence quotient, is simply a numerical score derived from a person's performance on one test (i.e., one set of items). The collection of items in any one test measures only a portion of the person's intelligence. Editorializing for the readers of *Saturday Review,* Woodring (1966) briefly described intelligence and the parts of intelligence measured by tests:

It is generally agreed that a person of high intelligence is one who can grasp ideas readily, make distinctions, reason logically, and make use of verbal and mathematical symbols in solving problems. An intelligence test is a rough measure of a child's capacity for learning, particularly for learning the kinds of things required in school. It does not measure character, social adjustment, physical stamina, manual skills, or artistic abilities. It is not supposed to—it was not designed for such purposes. To criticize it for such failure, is roughly comparable to criticizing a thermometer for not measuring humidity or wind velocity. (p. 6)

In describing how complex a concept intelligence is, Wechsler (1975) explained that intelligence, to

. . . the educator, . . . is most usefully defined as ability to learn; the biologist, as the ability to adapt; the psychologist, the ability to educe relationships; the computer programmer, as the facility to process information, etc. (p. 139)

However, regardless of how intelligence is defined, Strang (1958) pointed out that from the very beginning of life, intelligence,

. . . constantly creates itself by selecting, comparing, and organizing life experiences. Intelligence is not ready made, it is not passive; it does not merely respond to environmental pressures. It searches out experiences and inter-acts at the external environment. (p. 65)

The more intelligent individuals in a given situation profit more from that situation, and by that learning they are able to profit from the next situation more efficiently. In this way intelligence extends and elaborates itself. Unfortunately, many severely physically disabled children have less stimulating environments than average children, have fewer opportunities to interact with their environment, and as a result, their cognitive ability does not develop as rapidly as does cognitive ability in children of average physical ability.

Electricity is hard to define; but without knowing what it is, we can describe it in terms of ohms, amperes, and volts and measure what it does. Like electricity, intelligence is hard to define, but we can measure it well enough to know how much is there and ready to be plugged in.

According to Wechsler (1975),

Intelligence is an aspect of behavior; it has to do with appropriateness, effectiveness, and the worthwhileness of what human beings do or want to do . . . it is a many faceted entity, a complex of diverse and numerous components . . . it is not definable as a single trait or ability, (but) must be perceived as an overall or global capacity. (p. 135)

More intelligent individuals are able to function more efficiently than the less intelligent individuals. Such behavior is true within subcultures. While home and school experiences determine to a degree a person's opportunity to ascertain symbolic relationships, individuals with higher mental ability within a given environment use more symbols and recognize more important relationships among them than do individuals with lower ability (French, 1979).

Nonintellective Components of Intelligence

For decades Terman (1954) and Wechsler (1940) have referred to nonintellective factors of intelligence, such as drive, persistence, and goal awareness. In summarizing his longitudinal study of 1500 gifted individuals, both 20 and 30 years into the study, Terman concluded that tests of "general intelligence" given during the elementary school year predict a great deal about the ability to achieve, both in school at the time when tests are administered and 30 years later, but it was clear to Terman that mere intelligence was not enough. He recognized that both interest patterns and special aptitudes play important roles in achievement, for example, as a scientist, mechanic, author, artist, or mathematician. In comparing the most and least successful 150 men, he found the most successful to have more prudence, self-confidence, perseverance, desire to excel, goal-directed behavior, and freedom from inferiority feelings. The attributes which separated the most from the least successful men were those about which the environment at home and school have great influence. People with drive and persistence to attain a particular goal who do not have as high an IQ can match or exceed in performance persons with higher IQs but who have less interest in obtaining that goal.

These nonintellective but catalytic characteristics of individuals can be shaped. Without recognizing what they are doing, many parents of handicapped children and (mainstream) teachers become overprotective. Some authors (Blencowe, 1969; Cruickshank, 1976; Miller, 1958) attribute overprotective behavior to a sense of guilt and sympathy. Unfortunately, such behavior inhibits learning and adapting to new situations as the children are deprived of a stimulating environment in a manner not unlike children who are rejected and isolated. Children need opportunities to attempt intellectual tasks which are difficult for them.

In classrooms, particularly those in the mainstream where teachers have not been adequately prepared for physically disabled children, it is not uncommon to find cerebral palsied children receiving special privileges and teachers accepting academic performances that do not stretch the child. Psychologists also may be sympathetically biased when assessing cerebral palsied children. Psychologists may be reluctant to push passive, submissive children enough to obtain their maximum level of functioning.

Test Results and Client Variables

In administering tests, the examiner should observe carefully how the child deals with the questions and requests. Children who are attentive to the task, who are socially confident, who are eager to respond, who understand the directions and consider responses carefully, and who are willing to continue trying when puzzled or when failure is evident earn higher scores than those children who are playful or indifferent; who perform reluctantly or unwillingly; who are shy, apprehensive, or suspicious; who emphasize their inadequacies; who give up easily or attempt to change from difficult to easy tasks; who tire of the tasks quickly; and/or who react impulsively (French & Greer, 1965). In many test situations it is not clear whether the persons are able to exhibit more positive behaviors because they perceive themselves as having good ability; or whether because they have the more positive behaviors, they can earn higher scores. Scores for children who exhibit the behaviors associated with lower scores should be hypothesized to be underestimates of maximum ability. Higher IQs may be obtained when those children learn (or become able to exhibit) better test-taking skills such as those identified above (and others such as considering each request carefully, sitting quietly but responsively, etc.).

If intelligence tests are to be used successfully in measuring the maximum performance of an individual, the individual must be willing to provide maximum performance; and such willingness is usually based on an understanding (a) of why the behavior is requested, (b) of why it is important to perform it as well as possible, (c) that the person making the request be at least a reasonable (and preferably a friendly) person, and (d) that the individual has had some practice with activities similar to those required in that test condition. These variables influence test scores and must be considered by the psychologist responsible for the assessment. Children who respond reluctantly often earn scores lower than when they feel comfortable and want to do well.

Cultural Considerations

There is no doubt that intelligence tests, even when effectively administered, are culturally loaded. They are loaded toward middle America's expectations for school performance. Of course, a test can be culturally loaded but not be culturally biased. A test is not biased if scores from it predict the dependent variable (school success) equally well irrespective of group membership.

However, as Green (1959) has observed, many tests are biased because they reflect the curriculum of our schools and do not take into account the experiences of children from poor or minority families. We would add that they also fail to take into account the lack of experience resulting from restricted physical mobility. (See Cleary, Humphreys, Kendrick, and Wesman, 1975, for additional information about prediction of scholastic and job performance and Hunter and Schmidt, 1976, for a thoughtful analysis on the ethical use of tests.)

Intelligent behavior requires the capacity to perceive the situation correctly and to infer the consequences. A child may be better able to perceive the test situation correctly and infer more appropriately in some cultural settings than in others.

Learning and Intelligence

Persons who are skeptical about the value of intelligence tests often observe that verbal and numerical symbols can be taught, the ability to reason with them can be taught, and persistence and drive can be developed.

This is generally true; however, it is a mark of intelligence to discover independently the meaning of new symbols and the relationship between and among symbols. It requires less intellectual ability to have a teacher point out the relationships. With cerebral palsied children as with all children, the rate at which they learn is an important indicator of intelligence, as is their ability to bridge gaps to learn more than is taught. As problems are presented for which the answers or solutions have not been directly and consciously taught, psychologists can observe behavior from which intellectual level can be estimated. For these purposes the use of standardized, individually administered intelligence tests by well-prepared psychologists are essential in the assessment process.

What Intelligence Tests Measure

One of the founding fathers of American psychology said (more than 50 years ago) that intelligence is what intelligence tests measure. As the preceding section suggests, that often quoted simplistic comment is terribly misleading. Intelligence is far more than tests, even tests of today, measure. The matter is further complicated by the fact that some tests of intelligence measure some aspects of intelligence, and other tests measure other portions. Expressive vocabulary, receptive vocabulary, inductive reasoning, deductive reasoning, memory, spatial perception, speed of response, for example, are measured differentially by various tests. As a result, a score (or an IQ) from one test cannot be substituted for a score from another. Scores from different tests can be expected to be equivalent only to the extent that the content of the tests is the same. In selecting tests for use with cerebral palsied children it is essential to choose ones which measure as much of their cognitive ability and as little of their physical disability as possible. Of the many tests available, few were designed to allow such a distinction.

In a verbal society the size of one's receptive vocabulary and one's knowledge of basic symbols is a key item. Symbols in some common form must be employed to communicate with others and with one's self. Mere acquisition of symbols, however, is not sufficient. On the contrary, one must be able to relate symbols to each other, to discriminate among shades of meaning involving symbols that vary only slightly from one another and to perceive, to generalize, to synthesize, and to integrate. Newland (1962) refers to the symbols that are stored as *products* and the use of them to generalize, reason, and transfer as *process*. Cattell (1963) had a similar conceptualization but used as symbols the terms *crystalized* and *fluid* intelligence. By whatever term, the more intelligent in any group have more symbols and use them to solve problems more effectively than the less intelligent. To think and reason, one must have symbols. Whereas some reasoning requires spatial perception and/or symbols, verbal symbols are extremely important. The larger the vocabulary, the more symbols one has to use in reasoning.

As indicated above, cognitive ability develops; it does not appear full blown. The validity of cognitive ability scales for children are often indicated by observing older children earning higher raw scores than younger children. Older children have a larger vocabulary than those who are younger. Bright children of one age level have a larger vocabulary than average children. (Also, bright children use the symbols they have to reason better than other children.) In some scales, inappropriate for use with cerebral palsied children, items which require physical skill are included as indicators of cognitive ability (perhaps because they correlate well with cognitive abilities). In many infant scales we see developmentally ordered items as: holds head up, sits erect, walks, runs, skips. For older children we see items such as: draws a straight line at the three-year level of development, a circle at four years, a square at five, and a diamond at seven. Because the items are in a developmental order, we know that children who can draw a square can also draw a straight line and a circle. By observing that a child can draw a square, we need not ask him or her to draw a circle. We are justified in assuming that the child has the ability to draw a circle or a straight line if requested to do so. Because these drawing tasks are highly correlated with achievement in school, they appear in many school readiness tests. However, it is obvious that they are inappropriate for assessing the school readiness of cerebral palsied children. If they are used in this way, underestimates will occur.

To assess cerebral palsied children, we need items that indicate the level of development of mental or cognitive ability but require neither speech nor physical skill. In the first year of mental development children understand "no," indicate that they are hungry, make sounds to get attention, understand "bye-bye," anticipate uncovering of a toy, and differentiate between the voice of a familiar person and that of a stranger. Later they know names of frequently seen persons and objects; learn and follow rules; understand prepositions; and understand concepts such as tomorrow, yesterday, outside, far, and short. Because the developmental level of items can be determined for children, tests which include key or benchmark items can be used to estimate the level of mental development without trying to measure all that a child knows.

Scores from intelligence tests may be interpreted as measures of general mental ability but not as indices of achievement specifically taught in a common school curriculum. Although knowledge is required to answer items on intelligence tests, the items are selected to illustrate the ability to profit from exposure to learning in a variety of situations. High performance on the tests requires efficient utilization of verbal and numerical symbols, as well as the ability to retain information in symbol form for use at later times in the solution of verbal, quantitative, and abstract reasoning problems (French, 1964, 1979).

Scores from individually administered intelligence tests explain from about a quarter to half of the variability observed in scores from standardized achievement tests and a little less of the variability in teacher grades or ratings of academic performance (Sattler, 1974).

USE OF INTELLECTUAL ASSESSMENT
FOR PREDICTION AND PLANNING

Two important reasons for determining the cerebral palsied child's level of intellectual functioning are (a) to have a basis for predicting achievement, and (b) for planning educational programs.

Prediction

To predict whether an individual will profit appreciably from additional learning, the best predictor will be based on measures of previously acquired learning. Basically, intelligence tests have been designed to measure those aspects of mental ability that are important for success in school work. Scores from intelligence tests are not measures of innate capacity, but rather are based on learning experiences of the individual. Each bit of learning in turn predisposes the individual for learning additional responses, which enable him or her to display new acts of intelligent behavior. Intelligence tests include sets of standardized questions and tasks, which are used to determine one's accomplishments, for the prediction of learning in the educational mainstream. Because of this level of accomplishment within a fixed period of time, the tests also suggest an individual's potential for developing useful behavior in similar learning situations.

Predictive efficiency of some tests is reduced because they give points for speedy and correct responses. Others count the numbers of correct responses in a short period of time, but slowness is not equal to dullness even among physically able people. Although some life situations call for snap decisions and impulsive-like behavior, others call for reflection, careful consideration of each of several courses of action, and selection of the most appropriate response. In estimating the overall functional ability of a person, we need to measure both speedy responses and the quality of those obtained after reflection. With some tests it is not possible to determine the effect "speed of response" has in determining the total score. Scores from such tests must be used with extreme caution, especially when assessing children with neuromotor dysfunction.

Another factor which influences the predictive efficiency of intelligence tests is that IQs are not fixed. They do change both from test to test, as suggested above, and on the same test over time. Low IQs do not fluctuate as much over time as do high IQs. Generally, over a period of several years, a change as large as 15 points can be observed for one-fifth of the population (Reschly, 1979). A change of more than 15 points can be expected from a very small percentage of the population. Large changes are usually associated with significant changes in the environment or personal/social adjustment. Because such changes take place, an IQ obtained by a qualified examiner under good conditions should be interpreted as an indicator of current intellectual functioning. Since IQs do change, regular, thorough reevaluations are essential.

In the manual for the second edition of the Stanford-Binet test, Terman and Merrill (1937) warn that "abilities are always manifested and measured in relation to experience and training, and the behavioral composite which we call intelligence is of necessity modified and molded by these factors" (p. 65). In assessing one's intellectual potential, the score obtained from one test administration will not be sufficient for long-term predictions, particularly when the individual has recently enrolled in a more intensive educational and therapeutic environment. As an individual has more experiences in an interactive education (and is comfortable in it), the usefulness of one score may be improved; but as one is obtaining increased experience in such a setting, assessment of intellectual potential is best obtained from a series of measures over a period of time. Individuals whose IQs increase with repeated measurement over several years can be expected to be brighter than any of the scores indicate, and to be brighter than individuals of the same average IQ for whom progressively higher IQs on repeated measures were not noted. IQs of 60, then 70, then 80 have been observed for severely physically handicapped individuals who were assumed initially to be of below average intellectual ability. Because of their severe physical handicap and consequent lack of typical experiences in their first years of life, they were unable to earn higher scores on the tests which were administered. However, as the children profited from physical therapy and from a concentrated educational program, they were able to demonstrate more of the intellectual ability they possess. Similar observations have been made with bilingual children, whose scores improved as they became more adept in using the symbols of the cultural mainstream. The increasing scores did not indicate that the basic intelligence of the individual improved, but by being more able to communicate in the cultural mainstream, the rate of intellectual development appeared to improve. And because they could learn and manipulate the symbols used in the mainstream at an increasing rate, they were judged to be at least as bright as the last IQ would indicate as opposed to initial, lower IQs. Perhaps such individuals will continue to learn at a rate higher than indicated by the previous scores. Only time will tell.

Unfortunately, tests which minimize the physical disabilities of severely involved cerebral palsied children have not yet been developed for adolescents. As improved technology facilitates expression, this problem may be overcome.

IQs which are lower each time a measurement is made suggest that immediate attention be given to the cause. Is it physiological? Emotional? Educational? Can the trend be reversed?

Planning

The greatest value of standardized cognitive ability tests is in identification of the "present levels of educational performance" as required by PL 94-142 (U.S. Congress, 1975) for each student's "individualized educational program." Through the use of intelligence tests, psychologists can determine the general level of mental functioning, then select an appropriate broad-band (i.e., wide ranging) achievement test to get a more specific estimate of accomplishment in the basic skills. Achievement tests usually cover material recently taught from a designated curriculum, while intelligence tests sample a range of older and less deliberately acquired knowledge. Nationally standardized achievement test content is changed when it is clear that the curriculum of most schools is being changed. Intelligence tests, while containing some items that are specifically taught in school, are intended to be more general and require the additional use of intellectual processes. If the scores from the intelligence test are much higher than the norm referenced scores on the achievement test, it is clear that the individual is achieving less in school than in society in general; a remediation plan may be suggested. If the individual is out of the cultural mainstream or is in a restricted environment, even the intelligence score may be an underestimate of what it might be after a long period of intensive schooling.

If there is a need for further educational evaluation to assist in program planning, achievement tests with many items near the child's threshold for mastery can be administered to establish more accurate estimates of accomplishment in the basic skill areas. (See Salvia & Ysseldyke, 1978, Chapter 9.) Scores from standardized tests may be used in evaluating the effectiveness of procedures which have been used in the educational process. With these data as a base, annual goals and specific instructional objectives can be formulated, and the specific services to be provided can be identified as required by federal law; but beyond using the obtained scores for a status report about the child's level of function, information obtained in the data gathering process should be helpful in formulating interventions and instructional procedures (Bagnato & Neisworth, 1981). Reports are more helpful when they go beyond the test scores and test terminology to emphasize the qualitative features of a child's performance. By reporting about such things as "persistence, attention, organizational approach, speed of response, and need for feedback" (p. 13), readers of the report can determine the similarity between the child's performance in the testing situations in which they work. Also, such information can be helpful in setting goals.

FACTORS INFLUENCING
VALIDITY OF ASSESSMENT

When a test is administered to a child with cerebral palsy, it is expected that the score obtained will represent the child's ability in what the test purports to measure. Careful attention must be given to many factors to obtain the highest possible level of validity.

Test Selection and Interpretation

The importance of a thorough intellectual assessment of cerebral palsied children in developing appropriate educational programs for them has long been recognized (Doll, Phelps, & Melcher, 1932). A client-centered behavioral approach has been advocated by such persons as Bice (1948), Doll (1952), Haeussermann (1958), Michael-Smith (1955), and Taylor (1959). They have offered numerous suggestions for methods to improve psychological techniques for assessment. Use of tests which eliminate both verbalization and manipulation of objects by the child is most desirable. Who is to say that the cerebral palsied child, whose speech is only slightly affected, is able to respond orally as fully as he or she could if speech were not required. When oral responses are required with a test, we know that the child is at least as good as the score indicates or that when speech is required in a situation, the score is indicative of the child's functional level. Although numerous authors suggest modifying test items and using open-ended clinical evaluations, the value of the available normative data is lost. Only the subjective appraisal of the evaluator remains.

It is a common assumption among those engaged in intellectual assessment that when using a standardized instrument according to standard procedure, a psychologist will rarely, if ever, overestimate a child's abilities, and especially so if the child's experiential background is that of the norm group. In practice the interpretive trend has been to place less importance on the lower scores obtained and to use the higher scores as the more accurate indicators of the cerebral palsied child's mental ability (Berko, 1953). Research in recent years, however, has emphasized the need for a number of observations or sources of information for combination in a global score for reliable prediction of future learning. Differences in subtest scores are usually too unreliable to be meaningfully interpreted.

The *Pictorial Test of Intelligence* (PTI) (French, 1964) is composed of six subtests sampling a variety of intellectual functions. The items require neither speech, nor a fine motor response. To respond a child must have near normal visual and auditory acuity and must be able to indicate which of several drawings answer the examiner's request. Most children point to their answer with a hand movement, but some simply look at their choice. Most of the hundreds of cerebral palsied children I have tested with the PTI earn higher scores on the pictures vocabulary subtest than would be expected by their performance on the other subtests. The value of the PTI over other tests that measure only picture vocabulary (or spatial relationships) is that the PTI is comprised of six subtests each of which requires a different type of mental processing.

While a vocabulary test can provide a good estimate of general mental ability among average children in the mainstream culture, among cerebral palsied children the use of a picture vocabulary test only is an inadequate sample of general motor ability. Cerebral palsied children often earn higher scores on picture vocabulary tests than they do on tests requiring other aspects of intellectual ability. Items sampling other types of mental ability are essential for estimating the level of expected educational accomplishment.

Breen (1980) studied the verbal subtest data from Wechsler's scale for 93 cerebral palsied children enrolled in three residential centers. He found that, as anecdotal information from psychologists familiar with the cerebral palsied populations suggested, significantly higher scores were obtained for the sample on the similarities subtest, and significantly lower scores were obtained on the arithmetic subtest when the subtests were compared. Some would interpret these findings as indicating that these subjects need more education with numbers and numerical reasoning and that the reasoning required in answering the questions in the similarities subtests suggests a higher level of intellectual functioning than the verbal IQ would suggest. Whereas these may be tenable hypotheses, it is safer to conclude that the verbal IQ or the intellectual level based on each of the subtests, when combined with other observations from a variety of sources, is the best indication of a given child's general level of intellectual functioning.

To obtain the best scores from tests for interpretation, we must have complete, well-written manuals for use by personnel who have been adequately prepared in measurement theory and practice (Cegalka, 1978). The tests must be administered as they were standardized and the responses of subjects accurately evaluated in order for correct scores to be obtained (Sattler, 1974). Testing of cerebral palsied clients, therefore, requires careful test selection and interpretation. The Appendix contains brief descriptions of individually administered tests which are useful in whole or in part for assessing cerebral palsied children and adolescents.

Relationship Between Psychologist and Child

Scores from tests should reflect the best ability of each person. Much has been said about establishing an appropriate relationship between the psychologist and the subject before beginning formal evaluation. (See Sattler, 1974, pp. 71–76.)

When an examiner and a child first meet, it is necessary for them to become acquainted. When the examiner is a "familiar face" to the child, establishing an appropriate relationship for testing is relatively easy. Many examiners make it a point to be seen in classrooms and on the playground and to talk with various children in nontest situations to facilitate establishing rapport when testing takes place. Sometimes, small talk prior to entering the testing room and in the testing room is necessary; and in some cases, with a particularly apprehensive or uncooperative child, several nontesting activities may be necessary in the room to be used for testing before the actual administration of test items begins. By knowing what the child can do well in other situations, the examiner can often ask the child to do that for him in the test room as a warm-up function.

It is usually best to explain the kinds of activities expected in the test without referring to "games." Most children recognize that the test items are not games. Giving an example item or two and suggesting that most children like the activities is usually enough. A good explanation of the activities need not include the words "intelligence" or "test," if it is thought that those words will increase the child's anxiety.

Testing preschool children sometimes presents special problems because they have not yet learned to leave their parents for any length of time to be with another adult, no matter how pleasant the person may seem. While it is desirable to work alone with the child (without potential coaching from a parent), it is sometimes necessary for a parent to go along to the testing room. Should this become necessary, the parent's role must be explained in advance. In most instances, the parent will be able to sit behind the child, yet be in close enough physical proximity to give emotional support. A child on a mother's lap often receives kinesthetic clues which are difficult for the examiner to observe. Individuals who are old enough and intellectually able enough to know why they are responding to a test can have the testing situation explained to them sufficiently to elicit their best performance. (A psychologist should always be concerned about whether or not this has occurred, and should check with other persons to determine whether or not the performance is as can be reasonably expected.) For younger children it is not as easy to explain the importance of the activity. Therefore, an all-out effort must be made to ensure that the conditions under which the tests are administered will enable the child to pay attention to the requirements and to respond as efficiently as possible.

We all know that each child is unique, but individual differences among cerebral palsied children are even greater. Itinerant workers need help from those who work regularly with the child if they are to work effectively.

Awareness of Acuity and Perceptual Problems

Many cerebral palsied children are thought to have visual and/or auditory perceptual problems. It is probable that these perceptual problems are on a continuum, and only the gross problems are diagnosed with confidence. (See Chapters 5 and 6.) Children whose condition is not diagnosable may be disabled to the extent that sensory input is distorted enough to affect learning and, as a result, over time the ability to learn.

Psychologists need to know about visual and auditory acuity and perception, hand preference, and effective work space (i.e., right side, left side). Whereas such information may be in the child's records, consultation with teachers and therapists who work with the child on a regular basis can be helpful, as the following anecdote illustrates. A child who drooled was given a tissue to wipe up the saliva which accumulated during testing. I observed that he placed the tissue between the right eyelid and his glasses while I was giving a test requiring fine visual discrimination among geometric forms. Later, a therapist told me that whereas each eye was correctable to 20/20 as the records indicated, his binocular vision did not focus at near points. Had I known this before starting the testing, at the least, I could have had a larger supply of tissues.

Environment and Positioning

Room conditions are of considerable importance. The room should appear pleasant and be well lit, but without distracting stimuli. Ideally, the child should be familiar with the room and have pleasant associations with it. The child should be made as comfortable as possible. Only the materials used with the specific test items should be visible at one time. Other materials should be accessible to the examiner but out of sight and reach of the child. Furniture should be of appropriate size, so that the child's feet are on the floor and not dangling several inches above it. The table on which the test items are displayed should be low enough so that the child can view the material effectively and so that if manipulation of materials is necessary, it will be as easy as possible. If the client is to be tested in a wheelchair, a table which is both adjustable in height and which is large enough to display the materials is essential.

Eye contact by the examiner with the child is essential. In working with small children not best positioned in their own wheelchair, the examiner often needs to sit in a low chair, so that their heads are at about the same level. Consultation with a physical therapist about positioning is essential.

Time of Testing

Children should be tested at times when they have abundant energy, and at times when they are not concerned about missing something which to them is more important such as recess, storytime, or music. To be called away for testing while classmates are engaging in some more enjoyable activity may reduce the child's enthusiasm. Young children are usually more alert and receptive early in the morning or just after a recess or lunch break. Prescribed medicine affects children differently. Some are more efficient shortly after taking the drug, others at a midpoint between administrations, others as the effect is wearing off. Consultation with a teacher, therapist, or nurse about appropriate time and time limitations is essential. Tests which can be given easily to physically average children in one sitting often need to be divided into two or more sessions for cerebral palsied children for reasons associated with their condition.

Communication Between Psychologist and Child

It is essential that the psychologist use good voice projection and good articulation. Some children who are able to respond when they know what to do, are reluctant to ask for a question to be repeated or elaborated. With children who have a speech problem, it may be helpful to use a speech clinician to help record responses of the child. Such children should also have the opportunity to respond to tests that require no speech from them.

REFERENCES

Bagnato, S. J., & Neisworth, J. T. (1981). *Linking developmental assessment and curricula*. Rockville, MD: Aspen.

Berko, M. (1953). Some factors in the mental evaluation of cerebral palsy children. *Cerebral Palsy Review, 14*(5), 6–8.

Bice, H. (1948). Psychological examination of the cerebral palsied. *Exceptional Children, 14*, 163–168.

Blencowe, S. M. (1969). *Cerebral palsy and the young child*. Edinburgh: Earl S. Livingston Ltd.

Breen, J. P. (1980). *The performance of cerebral palsied children on the verbal subtests of the Wechsler Intelligence Scale*. Unpublished master's thesis, The Pennsylvania State University, University Park, PA.

Cattell, R. B. (1963). Theory of fluid and crystallized intelligence: A critical experiment. *Journal of Educational Psychology, 54*, 1–22.

Cegalka, W. (1978). Competencies of persons responsible for classification of mentally retarded persons. *Exceptional Children, 45*, 26–31.

Cleary, T. A., Humphreys, L. G., Kendrick, S. A., & Wesman, A. (1975). Educational uses of tests with disadvantaged populations. *American Psychologist, 30*, 15–41.

Cruickshank, W. (Ed.). (1976). *Cerebral palsy: A developmental disability*. Syracuse: Syracuse University Press.

Doll, E. (1952). Mental evaluation of children with cerebral palsy. *The Crippled Child, 39*(1), 6–7, 28.

Doll, E., Phelps, W., & Melcher, R. (1932). *Mental deficiencies due to birth injuries*. New York: Macmillan.

French, J. L. (1964). *Pictorial Test of Intelligence*. Boston: Houghton-Mifflin.

French, J. L. (1979). Intelligence: Its measurement and its relevance for education. *Professional Psychology, 10*, 753–759.

French, J. L., & Greer, D. R. (1965). Effect of test item arrangement on physiological and psychological behavior in primary school children. *Journal of Educational Measurement, 1*, 151–154.

Green, R. L. (1959). Tips on educational testing: What teachers and parents should know. *Phi Delta Kappan, 57*, 89–93.

Haeussermann, E. (1958). Evaluating the developmental level of cerebral palsy preschool children. *Journal of Genetic Psychology, 80*, 3–23.

Hunter, J., & Schmidt, F. (1976). Critical analysis of the statistical and ethical implications of various definitions of test bias. *Psychological Bulletin, 83*, 1053–1073.

Michael-Smith, H. (1955). Problems encountered in the psychometric examination of the child with cerebral palsy. *Cerebral Palsy Review, 16*(3), 15.

Miller, E. (1958). Cerebral palsied children and their parents. *Exceptional Children, 24*, 298–302; 305.

Newland, T. E. (1962). The assessment of exceptional children. In W. M. Cruickshank (Ed.), *Psychology of exceptional children and growth* (pp. 53–117). Englewood Cliffs, NJ: Prentice Hall.

Reschly, D. (1979). Nonbiased assessment. In G. Phye & D. Reschly (Eds.), *School psychology: Perspectives and issues* (pp. 215–254). New York: Academic Press.

Salvia, J., & Ysseldyke, J. E. (1978). *Assessment in special and remedial education*. Boston: Houghton-Mifflin.

Sattler, J. (1974). *Assessment of children's intelligence*. Philadelphia: E. B. Saunders.

Strang, R. (1958). The nature of giftedness. *Education of the gifted, The 57th yearbook of the National Society for the Study of Education: Part II* (pp. 64–86). Chicago: University of Chicago Press.

Taylor, E. (1959). *Psychological appraisal of children with cerebral defects.* Cambridge: Harvard Press.

Terman, L. M. (1954). The discovery and encouragement of exceptional talent. *American Psychologist, 9,* 221–230.

Terman, L. M., & Merrill, M. A. (1937). *Measuring intelligence.* Boston: Houghton-Mifflin.

U.S. Congress. (1975). Federal Public Service 94-142. *Congressional Record,* 94th Congress, November 29, *12,* 773–796.

Wechsler, D. (1940). Nonintellective factors in general intelligence. *Psychological Bulletin, 37,* 444–445.

Wechsler, D. (1975). Intelligence defined and undefined: A relativistic appraisal. *American Psychologist, 30,* 135–139.

Woodring, P. (1966). Are intelligence tests unfair? *Saturday Review, 49,* 79–80.

CHAPTER 4

Social and Emotional Development

Eugene T. McDonald

*McDonald contends that, at all developmental stages, program-
ming for persons with cerebral palsy must focus on social-
emotional problems along with physical, cognitive, and medical problems.*

1. *What is the evidence that social-emotional problems occur
   frequently in cerebral palsy, and what causes have been
   proposed to explain the linkage?*
2. *Describe how important aspects of social-emotional
   development in infancy are adversely affected by the neuromuscular dysfunction of cerebral palsy.*
3. *How do self-concept and social competency emerge during
   early childhood, and how is their development often
   thwarted in cerebral palsy?*
4. *What are the main areas of social-emotional development
   during middle childhood? How do the neuromuscular
   dysfunction and associated problems of cerebral palsy
   interfere with social-emotional development during this
   period?*
5. *Adolescence, as a time of transition between childhood
   and adulthood, is marked by internal and external
   changes. What are the important changes, and how are
   they affected by cerebral palsy?*

INTRODUCTION

Social and emotional development have not been studied as systematically as cognitive and physical development. Conner, Williamson, and Siepp (1978) concluded, "Except for some good research on the development of attachment, little work has been focused on the sequential development of social skills or emotional patterns." They suggest the available studies tend to be narrow in scope. Participants in a recent conference on facilitating social-emotional development in young multiply-handicapped children noted a lack of supportable theories about early social-emotional development (McDonald & Gallagher, 1984). Writing about affective education for special children and youth, Morse, Ardizzone, Macdonald, and Pasik (1980) said there is little reasonable theory about the nature and purpose of affective education and note that the field has been called "chaotic and unorganized." Even though research and theory development in this area are not far advanced, there is evidence to indicate that children born with cerebral palsy are at high risk for social-emotional development. In this chapter we will identify risk factors at several developmental periods.

INDICATIONS OF DEVELOPMENTAL FACTORS

There is evidence from a variety of sources that many persons with cerebral palsy exhibit signs of emotional immaturity and social maladjustment.

Teachers, therapists, and other professional personnel often comment about the social-emotional immaturity of the cerebral palsied individuals with whom they work. Commonly, in written reports and conferences, they describe many children as taking little part in activities. Their passivity is observed in self-help as well as in social and educational activities. Older children are often seen as having settled into the role of a passive recipient of care. Teachers and therapists frequently feel that lack of progress in education or development of physical skills is due to lack of motivation. Such children seem not to develop the normal drive to try new things or to work at a task until it is mastered. Another frequent observation is that many children with cerebral palsy are lacking in social awareness. By this, observers seem to mean that the children are egocentric rather than sociocentric in their orientation. This focus on self, however, is not accompanied by a favorable self-concept or high self-esteem. Some children give the impression of being emotionless, seldom showing signs of such feelings as happiness, sadness, or anger. Of course, not all children with cerebral palsy are so described, but unfortunately the social-emotional status of many, especially those who are severely involved, is described in such terms as "passive," "unmotivated," "lacking in social awareness," "poor self-image," and "emotionless." Obviously, these are subjective evaluations, but the frequency with which they are made by teachers, therapists, and other professional workers strongly suggests that many persons with cerebral palsy experience difficulty in areas of social-emotional development.

In their review of studies of emotional disturbance in cerebral palsy, Hourcade and Parette (1984) found "a consistent overrepresentation of emotional disturbances" in persons with cerebral palsy. They note that three causes have been proposed: direct effects of CNS pathology, secondary problems associated with the motor handicap, and distorted parent-child interactions. Phelps' (1948) view that certain social-emotional characteristics are associated with specific types of cerebral palsy strongly influenced the early thinking of professional workers. He contended that each of the major types of cerebral palsy has a unique set of personality characteristics. The differences were held to be so noticeable that a diagnosis of the physical condition could be made almost by observing the social-emotional characteristics. For example, spastics were described as introverted, fearful, slow to anger, and as preferring verbal expressions of pity to demonstrations of love. Athetoids, on the other hand, were thought to be extroverted, fearless, quick to anger, and as enjoying expressions of love and affection. When professional workers were asked to describe the social-emotional characteristics of individual cerebral palsied children it was found that effective predictions of the behavior in terms of love, anger, and fear responses could not be made on the basis of type of cerebral palsy (Garmezy, 1953). However, it was found in this study that emotional immaturity and overdependency were frequently observed. Garmezy suggested, "It would not be an untoward assumption that the social and familial milieu of the child may exercise an important role in the determination of his emotional and social behavior."

Many adults with cerebral palsy exhibit social-emotional difficulties which adversely affect their coping abilities. Glick (1953) reported that 75% of cerebral palsied adults who had applied for assistance in finding employment exhibited behavior indicative of poor social-emotional adjustment which in 20% was severe enough to preclude job placement. Among the feelings and attitudes identified by interviewers were unrealistic attitudes, intense feeling of insecurity, extreme immaturity, excessive fears, strong feelings of inferiority, low frustration tolerance, problems in interpersonal relationships, and lack of motivation. Later studies (Jones & Maschmeyer, 1958; Minde, 1978; Storrow & Jones, 1960) have reported a high percentage of social-emotional difficulties in adolescents and adults. Freeman (1970) suggests that the social-emotional problems manifested in adolescence are the result of the interaction of several etiological factors. The onset of many of these problems can be traced to experiences during infancy and early childhood.

SOCIAL–EMOTIONAL DEVELOPMENT IN INFANCY

Infants begin interacting with persons and things at birth. The nature of these interactions influences the child's social-emotional development. Even at this early age, interactions are complex and intervening variables numerous, making it difficult to conduct controlled investigations (Siegel, 1982). However, enough has been learned to suggest some possible origins of the social-emotional problems seen in cerebral palsy. Many factors which stimulate and direct social-emotional development operate abnormally in children with neurodevelopmental problems.

Bonding

It has been hypothesized that early and extended physical contact between the mother and newborn infant establishes a bond which will positively affect the later behaviors of both mother and infant. Further, it is speculated that a physiological readiness for bonding may exist in the mother for a few days after giving birth. To capitalize on this readiness, skin-to-skin contact with suckling following delivery is practiced in some hospitals and there is experimentation with periods of "rooming-in" during which the mother and newborn have extended contact. In these programs mothers are seen to exhibit increased eye-to-eye contact, smiling, kissing, singing, and other types of vocalization and the infants are reported to be more responsive and alert. The long-range effects of bonding are not clear; however, it is plausible to expect that they will be positive. Infants born prematurely, who suffer birth trauma, or who for other reasons are at risk—conditions which may result in cerebral palsy—are often deprived of positive bonding experiences.

Attachment

Establishment of a two-way attachment between infant and caregiver (usually the mother) constitutes an important base for social and emotional development. Both mother and infant make contributions to the interaction. Attachment progresses through a series of cues and responses. For example, the baby's crying gets the mother's attention and she picks up her child. Baby responds by cuddling or molding, and mother provides care and loving; baby becomes quiet. At each step, baby and mother provide positive reinforcement for the other's behavior. Normally each sensory modality is stimulated by the presence and behavior of mother and infant and contributes to the characteristics of the attachment which is formed.

The sensations associated with feeding and holding strengthen the relationship between mother and child. Eye contact begins early and is an important step toward development of the social smiling which so powerfully influences maternal behavior. Bouncing and other types of playing give rise to pleasant tactile and movement sensations. The mother's voice alerts the baby and provokes smiles, and mothers, in turn, are fascinated by their infants' noncrying vocalizations. During the first year these interactive behaviors build a special relationship between the child and caretakers.

The nature of attachment is dynamic. Until about 6 months of age, most infants respond to attention from almost anyone, including strangers. During the second half-year, infants tend to resist being handled by anyone except their primary caregiver. During the second year, while maintaining a strong preference for their major caregiver, young children accept more readily the attention of a few other people with whom they are familiar.

Types of Attachment. There are differences in the types of attachment established. Most babies in middle-class families develop secure attachments to their mothers. Securely attached babies handle separation from their mothers with a minimum of fussing. Later they are willing to leave their mothers as they explore their environments using the mother as a safe base. Babies, who for various reasons have little close bodily contact and are otherwise handled ineptly by their mothers, are likely to be insecurely attached. Their behavior tends to clinging and weeping. They stay near their mothers and are less likely to engage in exploratory behavior. Follow-up studies suggest that early patterns of attachment are related not only to the child's relation with others but also to language and cognitive development (Ainsworth, 1982).

Effect of Neuromuscular Dysfunction. Crying, feeding, gazing and following, cuddling, smiling and vocalizing—the infant behaviors involved in attachment—require neuromuscular activity. Even these simple acts may be affected by the neuromotor dysfunction of cerebral palsy. The crying of some children has a peculiar sound and arouses maternal anxiety. Poor coordination makes nursing difficult for mother and baby, leading to feelings of frustration and sometimes guilt in the mother who blames herself for being unable to feed her baby. Cuddling in which the child's body is molded to conform to the mother's body is difficult for the baby with abnormal muscle tone. Children with abnormal tone may be difficult to pick up and handle for diapering and bathing, and play is discouraged. Attempts to smile might produce a grimace rather than the happy face by which babies enchant caregivers. Vocalizing is often delayed or abnormal in severely handicapped children. Mother-infant interactions are often stressful, and the experiences are not conducive to the formation of a secure attachment.

Awareness of Self

In the 1980 Nebraska Symposium on Motivation, Posner and Rothbart (1981) expressed the view that "of all categories learned by the infant perhaps the most crucial and the most difficult to understand is the category of self." Piaget (1967) regarded self-concept as basic to all other concepts the child acquires. Awareness of self as distinct from other people or objects in the environment is probably the first step toward development of a self-concept. When infants become aware of self is not known. Some theorists believe that infants are predesigned to make some primitive distinction between self and others (Stern, 1982) but other theorists hold the view that the newborn does not understand that there is any difference between self and others (Conner et al., 1978).

Normal Development. Awareness of self develops gradually. Experiences such as mouthing a fist, sucking a thumb, visually regarding a hand, touching a toy, touching another person, and being touched by another person develop a distinction between self and not-self. Social smiling and response to tickling are early signs of self-awareness. Smiling is often observed in 6-week-old babies, and by the end of the second month babies will smile in response to almost anyone. It appears that the baby is smiling *at* the other person. At about 3½ months of age, babies laugh out loud in resonse to tickling. White (1975) has suggested that tickling results in laughter only when the person tickled perceives that another person is producing the stimulation. Crawling produces many opportunities for discovery of self. A crawling baby can physically separate itself from mother, thus sharpening the distinction between self and others. As new environments are explored, the infant receives stimulation from external sources which further the differentiation between self and non-self. Though infants as young as 2 months are fascinated by their faces reflected in mirrors, signs of self-recognition do not appear until about 18 months. Self-awareness is a logical precursor to self-recognition. The later-developed verbal expressions of "me" and "mine" have their roots in awareness of self and clear distinction between what is self and what is not self, such as other people and objects in the environment.

Effect of Neuromuscular Dysfunction. There are no empirical data regarding development of self-awareness in children with cerebral palsy, but consideration of the normal process suggests several reasons why these children might need help in learning to differentiate self from others or from objects. Oculomotor dysfunction might make it difficult for the infant to fixate a gaze on the caretaker's face and to make the eye contact which Freedman (1965) considers important for development of social smiling. Social smiling elicits caretaker behavior which contributes to the infant's differentiation between self and others. Smiling may be delayed because of visual problems or poorly performed because of poor control of facial muscles. Children whose neuromuscular dysfunction interferes with respiration and phonation have difficulty laughing out loud and, hence, caretakers may not be encouraged to tickle them or play games which lead to self-awareness. Children who are hypersensitive to tactile stimulation may respond abnormally to tickling and thus discourage this activity. When infants cannot crawl, they are deprived of opportunities to learn about the self by physically separating themselves from others.

It is clear that infants with cerebral palsy are at risk for social-emotional development. Their neuromuscular dysfunction directly affects their own behavior, which in turn often adversely affects the attitudes, feelings, and behavior of parents who are usually the primary caretakers. The conditions produce a milieu which is less than optimal for social-emotional development.

SOCIAL–EMOTIONAL DEVELOPMENT OF EARLY CHILDHOOD

In normally developing children, the period following infancy is marked by rapid development of self-concept and social competency. These attributes are basic to other aspects of social-emotional development.

Self-Concept

How one views one's self is a powerful determinant of how one fits into the socio-economic life of our culture. One's view of self may change as one ages, but its roots are in early childhood experiences. Several factors influence the early development of self-concept.

Control Over Contingencies.   At an early age, normally developing children begin noting that their actions can influence events (e.g., a cry brings a caretaker, when a hand strikes a toy, the toy moves). Gradually, children become aware of what actions yield what outcomes, and they develop a rudimentary concept of cause-effect relationships. Positive feelings toward self are generated by successful attempts to exert some control over the environment. Each success seems to motivate the child to initiate actions appropriate to produce desired outcomes. On the other hand, when motor dysfunction results in unsuccessful attempts at control, positive feelings about self are not generated, and repeated failures weaken the motivation to continue trying.

Development of Independence.   Learning to carry out an act or to perform a task without help gives a powerful boost to self-esteem at all ages. A newborn is totally dependent on caretakers. For example, the feeding bottle must be held by another person and the nipple placed in the child's mouth. For change in position or movement from one place to another, the infant is also dependent on others. With maturation of neuro-muscular function, the child learns to handle the bottle alone. Develop-ment of unsupported sitting and upper extremity control frees the child from dependence on caretakers for getting food into the mouth. A walk-ing child is free to move about, no longer dependent on being carried to get a change of scene, and no longer having to wait for someone to get a toy. As time passes the child grows in awareness of body control—arms and hands, trunks and legs and, while still in early childhood, bowels and bladder. With each increment in level of independence the child's level of self-regard rises, making for stronger positive feelings toward self.

The shift from dependence to independence is closely related to develop-ment of neuromuscular control. Such control develops slowly and imper-fectly in some children with cerebral palsy, with adverse effects on development of a positive self-concept. Some, even into adulthood, remain dependent on caretakers in all activities of daily living. The negative effects of such dependence on self-concept are difficult to counteract.

Success in Communication. Learning to talk provides the develop-ing child with another powerful tool for exerting control. A simple action, producing spoken words, may be used in a variety of situations to yield many outcomes. "Mama" brings mother, "da" brings doll, milk may follow the utterance of "mu," and "bye" earns a trip outside. Language develop-ment has far-reaching implications for all aspects of social-emotional development as well as for cognitive development. Especially, self-concept is enhanced by the pleasure derived from acquisition of knowledge and expression of thoughts and feelings through communication.

Children who cannot learn to talk intelligibly and who have not devel-oped another adequate means of communication fail in their efforts to exer-cise control over their environments and to relate to others through communication. Repeated successes generate positive feelings of personal worth, whereas repeated failures result in negative feelings about self.

Reactions of Others. How we feel about ourselves is to a large extent determined by our perception of how others feel about us. Caplan and Caplan (1977) observed that among the earliest experiences that influence the development of a child's view of himself are those with other people, especially with the significant people in his life (at first, the parents or another primary caretaker). If children are accepted, respected, and liked for what they are, they will be helped immeasurably toward a healthy atti-tude of respect for themselves.

It is usually easy for the family to make normally developing children feel "accepted, respected and liked for what they are"; however, many fac-tors operate to interfere with the development of such a nurturing social-emotional climate for children severely handicapped by cerebral palsy. No parents choose to produce a handicapped child. Their dream is to have a child who will learn to walk, talk, carry out the activities of daily living, become educated, get a good job, marry, and have children. Awareness that their cerebral palsied child will not fulfill this dream naturally results in emotional stresses within the family. Added to these emotional strains are others arising from uncertainties about how to handle the child, fatigue from the constant care required, and conflicts among family members about the nature of the child's problem—what caused it, who is to blame, and what should be done about it. It has been suggested that parents of handicapped children go through a period of mourning and grief similar to that associated with the death of a loved one (Tanner, 1980). There is, however, a major difference. Death removes the loved one, and with the passage of time grief loses its poignancy. Cerebral palsied children live on, and the impact of their handicap becomes more apparent with the passage of time. Parents expect to feed, bathe, dress, and care for the toilet needs of infants. To realize that they must provide such care through childhood—and perhaps throughout the child's life—is emotionally disturbing to many parents. Parent-child interactions are bound to suffer in this emotional climate.

Social Competency

Social competency is a complex developmental process, consisting of knowledge, attitudes, and skills. Its characteristics change with time. What makes for social competence in childhood would be regarded as social incompetence in an adolescent, and appropriate adolescent social behavior would be inappropriate in adults. Some changes, however, are merely elaborations or refinements of knowledge, attitudes, and skills which individuals begin acquiring in early childhood.

Adjusting to Different Situations. Separation from mother—secure in the knowledge that the separation is only temporary—is an early step in developing social competence. Through play, preschool children learn to feel comfortable even when mother is not present. At first, children play independently with toys but not with other children even when they are together; but, by age 3, most children play cooperatively with others—even sharing toys. By age 4, most children prefer group to independent play and, by age 5, they can work cooperatively with several other children in carrying out a project such as building a house of blocks. Not only are they learning to interact with others, they are also learning how to act when in new places and engaged in a variety of activities.

Learning Rules and Developing Attitudes. Socialization is the process of learning the rules of behavior for a given social group and acquiring the motivation to perform properly. Children learn the rules largely by observation, experience, and some parental teaching. As they play "doctor," "school," "house," or "tea party," children verbalize the rules of behavior in these situations and are motivated to follow the rules. Role playing and pretend play also help children become aware of the emotions of others (Chance, 1979).

In the normally developing child, play typically involves motor activity and communication. Children, who because of their motor dysfunction cannot move about or communicate easily with other children, have difficulty in joining a social group and learning its rules of behavior.

Learning to Control Emotions and Express Feelings.   Socially competent persons can govern their emotions and express their feelings in socially acceptable ways. Emotional control develops gradually. The uncontrolled anger and frustration of young children often results in a tantrum with screaming and excessive physical action such as kicking, hitting, falling on the floor, and headbanging. As children mature, such extreme behavior is brought under control; however, until about age 7 children "express emotions primarily through their bodies and not through words" (Morse et al., 1980). Parents and others learn to interpret the child's physical actions—a form of body language—as cues to a variety of feelings. Social competence requires that emotionally toned words, as well as actions, be controlled. Children learn that joyous outbursts may be appropriate in some situations but not others. There is a time and place for speaking of love. Unrestrained venting of anger and hostility rarely, if ever, is socially acceptable. Through interaction with peers and observation of adults in a variety of situations, children gradually become knowledgeable about what are and what are not appropriate verbal or physical expressions of emotion. Maintaining emotional control is a process which begins in childhood, suffers setbacks during adolescence, and remains a challenge throughout life.

Many cerebral palsied children are unable to use their bodies effectively to express emotions. They cannot show disapproval or anger by running away. Their body language is often difficult to read. Speech problems interfere with verbal expression of emotions, and opportunities to observe peers and adults are limited.

SOCIAL–EMOTIONAL DEVELOPMENT IN MIDDLE CHILDHOOD

The social-emotional developmental tasks of middle childhood are many, and some are especially difficult for the child with severe neuromuscular dysfunction.

Acquiring Increasing Amounts of Autonomy

Normally developing children gradually become more and more self-directing. They enjoy increasing independence in making decisions and in planning and carrying out activities. Parents extend privileges and help the child assume responsibilities leading eventually to functioning independently without control of others. During this period the child spends more and more time away from parents learning about the self and developing social skills. Parental discipline and control diminish as the child requires less physical care and supervision. Along with growing autonomy, the normally developing child develops controls which are essential for achieving a balance between personal desires and the kind of behavior required for acceptance by others.

Development of Peer Relationships

The peer group is a powerful determiner of behavior—often more so than family or school. True social interest in peers begins to emerge in the third year of life (White, 1975). Need for membership in a peer group becomes strong during the early school years. Peer groups are composed of individuals of similar status—persons who have much in common and can share experiences as equals. Acceptance by a peer group enhances the child's self-esteem, and identification with a group aids in developing a personal identity. The complex social relationships of peer groups provide opportunities to experience love-hate, cooperation-competition, acceptance-rejection, and many other feelings and attitudes. The social-emotional coping skills of the adult are in part shaped by the peer group experiences of childhood.

Broadening of Interests and Activities

While ties with home and family remain strong in middle childhood, other adults become important to the child as children of this age become increasingly involved in activities which take place outside the home. The play of earlier developmental stages gives way to sports, gangs, and clubs. During this period, children seem to thirst for new experiences. They try something for a short time only to give it up for something else. As children progress through middle childhood, they experience a growing need for opportunities for creative thinking and creative expression. Through participation in a variety of activities they can test themselves and evaluate their performances. They begin to learn what they can do well and what they do poorly, what they like and do not like, what brings them favorable attention and acceptance, and what leads to unfavorable attention and possible rejection. The interests and activities of this period are powerful influences on sense of self and one's feelings of self-esteem.

Cerebral Palsy and Middle Childhood

The neuromuscular dysfunction and associated problems of cerebral palsy interfere with the social-emotional development of this period. This is especially true for those who are nonambulatory and who have poor arm and hand function. Instead of learning to function independently without control of others, they remain dependent on others. Autonomy is unattainable for them or they can attain only a low level of autonomy. It is difficult for them to develop the peer relationships which are important to social-emotional growth because they cannot participate in the activities of their peers. Music lessons, sports, gangs, and clubs are not open to many children with cerebral palsy. Normal children have difficulty interacting with physically disabled children (Richardson, 1969); thus, opportunities for learning through peer relationships are reduced. Socialization under these circumstances is difficult.

SOCIAL–EMOTIONAL DEVELOPMENT IN ADOLESCENCE

It would be impossible to cover adequately the social-emotional development of adolescence in this short discussion. For a more detailed discussion, the reader is referred to a 1983 publication of the United Cerebral Palsy Association titled "Programming for Adolescents with Cerebral Palsy and Related Disabilities."[1] The following brief description of selected aspects of development in the nondisabled will call attention to the developmental problems of the disabled.

Physical

Adolescence is the period between the end of childhood and the beginning of adulthood. From the onset of puberty, body changes occur quickly. Height and weight increase, motor skills advance, and the individual becomes stronger. Secondary sex characteristics appear. Male voices change, pubic and facial hair appear. Boys become able to ejaculate. Girls develop breasts and begin to menstruate. In both sexes there is an upsurge of sexual feeling. Internal changes which affect physical growth and sexual maturation are also regarded as related to the adolescents' abrupt changes in mood and feelings.

Psychological

The adolescent is concerned with many processes which are affective in nature. The following are of particular importance for the adolescent with cerebral palsy.

---

[1] Available from United Cerebral Palsy Associations, Inc., 66 East 34 Street, New York, NY 10016.

Achieving Independence. Adolescents tend to be preoccupied by some formulation of such questions as "Who am I," "What are my values." Resolution of what has been called an "identity crisis" is achieved as the individual interacts with family, peers, and other members of society; considers and rejects ideas; tries and discards values. By late adolescence most individuals have developed a stable identity and system of values which prepare them to cope with the world as adults.

Preparing for an Occupation. During the early teen years both boys and girls are strongly motivated to earn some money of their own. They babysit, deliver newspapers, mow lawns, and take on a variety of odd jobs. Later many seek out steady part-time jobs where they work after school, on weekends, or during school vacations. Through these experiences, adolescents develop work habits and learn about what kind of work they might enjoy as adults. In later adolescence they become preoccupied with concerns about how they will earn a living. They seek full-time employment or enter education and training programs designed to prepare them for a vocation. They realize that being gainfully employed is essential in adulthood.

Sexuality

Sexuality, a dominant theme in adolescent development, is influenced by physical and psychological factors. The sexual awakening of early adolescence grows into the urgent sexual drives of later adolescence. The drives lead to social experiences which help shape the mature sexuality of the adult. The concept of sexuality includes, but is broader than, today's use of the word "sex." Cook (1983) defines sexuality as "one's sense of maleness or femaleness resulting from the integration of one's spiritual, intellectual, emotional, physical and socio-cultural aspects of human character at any point in time." Until recently sexuality in handicapped persons has been largely ignored or consideration was dominated by misconceptions. Sexuality is a universal characteristic of humans including those disabled by cerebral palsy.

Potential Effects of Cerebral Palsy

All aspects of social-emotional development pose difficulties for adolescents with cerebral palsy, especially those who are moderately or severely impaired. Their striving for autonomy is impeded or thwarted by their inability to carry out independently the activities of daily living. Their increase in height and weight adds to their caretaker's problems in dressing, feeding, bathing, and toileting. The personal identity they find is disappointing because the positive aspects may seem less important to them than the negative effect of their disabling physical condition. The natural desire to become gainfully employed and earn a living is difficult to fulfill. Failure of others to recognize their growing sexuality and their inability to find expression for their natural sexual urges is frustrating for the disabled adolescent. Some persons with cerebral palsy effectively cope with the risks to achieving satisfying social-emotional development. Many do not. For some, social-emotional problems are as handicapping as the physical condition.

IMPLICATIONS FOR PROGRAMMING

Persons with cerebral palsy are at high risk for social-emotional development. At every stage from infancy into adulthood factors related to the physical and associated problems of their condition interfere with normal social-emotional developmental processes. Unfortunately, most treatment programs have focused on physical, cognitive, and medical problems to the neglect of programs designed to enhance social-emotional development. It is imperative that techniques designed to facilitate social-emotional development be an integral part of every stage of the management program.

Parents of high risk infants need guidance and support so effective bonding and attachment can occur. Young cerebral palsied children need understanding and patient assistance as they try to influence events by communication and physical actions. Caretakers and professional workers must develop and use many ways to help the child develop a positive self-concept. The potentially detrimental attitudes and feelings which naturally arise in parents of handicapped children must be recognized, understood, and handled before they interfere with the child's social-emotional development. Special programs must be designed to help cerebral palsied children gain the experience which nonhandicapped children find in play and peer group activities. Attitudes of protectiveness and pity must give way to ongoing efforts to help the cerebral palsied individual gain the highest possible level of autonomy. Work opportunities must be developed for cerebral palsied persons, and they must be adequately prepared to take advantage of these opportunities. Social situations should be structured to encourage sexual development and allow for its expression.

The magnitude of the task of facilitating social-emotional development is overwhelming. Only through the interest and effort of all who work with the cerebral palsied can an effective program be initiated and conducted. Parents, physicians, psychologists, teachers, therapists, and administrative personnel must recognize that in addition to their specific responsibility they have a general responsibility to overcome the barriers to social-emotional development. Overcoming barriers does not always mean functioning in the mainstream of socioeconomic life; mainstreaming may not be possible or advisable for some persons with severe dysfunction. For them, programs must be developed which allow them to live, socialize, and work with handicapped peers.

REFERENCES

Ainsworth, M. D. S. (1982). Early caregiving and later patterns of attachment. *Birth, interaction and attachment.* Pediatric Round Table 6, Johnson and Johnson Baby Products.

Caplan, F., & Caplan, T. (1977). *The second twelve months of life.* New York: Grosset and Dunlap.

Chance, P. (1979). *Learning through play* (Summary of a Pediatric Round Table). New York: Garden Press, Inc.

Conner, F. P., Williamson, G. G., & Siepp, J. M. (1978). *Program guide for infants and toddlers with neurodevelopmental and other developmental disabilities.* New York: Teachers College Press.

Cook, R. N. (1983). Sexuality: Issues, perspectives, and guidelines. *Programming for adolescents with cerebral palsy and related disabilities.* New York: United Cerebral Palsy Associations, Inc.

Freedman, D. C. (1965). Hereditary control of early social behavior. In B. M. Foss (Ed.), *Determinants of infant behavior* (Vol. 3) (pp. 149–159). London: Methuen & Co. LTD.

Freeman, R. D. (1970). Psychiatric problems in adolescents with cerebral palsy. *Developmental Medicine and Child Neurology, 12,* 64–70.

Garmezy, N. (1953). Some problems with psychological research in cerebral palsy. *American Journal of Physical Medicine, 32,* 348–355.

Glick, S. J. (1953). Emotional problems in 200 cerebral palsied adults. *Cerebral Palsy Review, 14,* 3–5.

Hourcade, J., & Parette, H. P. (1984). Cerebral palsy and emotional disturbance: A review and implications for intervention. *Journal of Rehabilitation, 50,* 55–60.

Jones, M., & Maschmeyer, J. E. (1958). Childhood aims and adult accomplishments in cerebral palsy. *International Record of Medicine, 171,* 219–224.

McDonald, E. T., & Gallagher, D. L. (Eds.). (1984). *Facilitating social-emotional development in young multiply handicapped children: proceedings of a conference.* Philadelphia: Home of the Merciful Saviour.

Minde, K. K. (1978). Coping styles of 34 adolescents with cerebral palsy. *American Journal of Psychiatry, 135,* 1344–1348.

Morse, W. C., Ardizzone, J., Macdonald, C., & Pasik, P. (1980). *Affective education for special children and youth.* Reston, VA: The Council for Exceptional Children.

Phelps, W. M. (1948). Characteristic psychological variations in cerebral palsy. *Nervous Child, 7,* 10–13.

Piaget, J. (1967). *Six psychological studies.* New York: Random House.

Posner, M. I., & Rothbart, M. K. (1981). The development of attentional mechanisms. *1980 Nebraska symposium on motivation.* Lincoln: University of Nebraska Press.

Richardson, S. A. (1969). The effects of physical disability on the socialization of the child. In D. A. Goslin (Ed.), *Handbook of socialization theory and research.* Chicago: Rand McNally.

Siegel, E. (1982). A critical examination of studies of parent-infant bonding. *Birth, interaction and attachment.* Pediatric Round Table 6, Johnson and Johnson Baby Products.

Stern, D. (1982). Mothers and infants: The early transmission of affect. *Birth, interaction and attachment*. Pediatric Round Table 6, Johnson and Johnson Baby Products.

Storrow, H. A., & Jones, M. H. (1960). Management of emotional barriers to rehabilitation in cerebral palsied adults. *Archives of Physical Medicine and Rehabilitation, 41*, 570–574.

Tanner, D. C. (1980). Loss and grief: Implications for the speech language pathologist and audiologist. *ASHA, 22, 11*, 916–928.

White, B. L. (1975). *The first three years of life*. New York: Avon Books.

CHAPTER 5

Auditory Problems

Bruce M. Siegenthaler

The author presents an overview of the development and functioning of the auditory system and how it may be defective in children with cerebral palsy. Methods are described for assessing hearing function in children of various ages, with or without cerebral palsy, and some guidelines for interpreting auditory test data are provided.

1. What can we say about the comparative incidence of hearing loss among normal and cerebral palsied children?

2. What are the major divisions of the auditory system, and what does each contribute to overall hearing behavior or function?

3. What are the results of specific defects in specific parts of the auditory system?

4. How are hearing assessment procedures adapted for (a) ages of children, and (b) normal versus cerebral palsied children?

5. Make a list or catalog of audiological tests (be sure to include behavioral observations) and contrast the responses of normal versus hearing impaired cerebral palsied children.

6. Expand the list of the other sources, in the form of an annotated bibliography of at least 10 more items, on the topic of remedial or training procedures applicable to the hearing impaired cerebral palsied child.

INTRODUCTION

Assessing the hearing of cerebral palsied persons is a challenge. Especially among younger cerebral palsied children, lack of response may be interpreted as deafness even though there is no hearing loss. Pennsylvania Department of Health records show the incidence of hearing loss in school children to be between 2½% and 3%. Although the data shown in Table 5.1 have high variability, various classifications and sample sizes of cerebral palsy, and although the validity of specific studies is not evaluated, it seems evident that the incidence of hearing loss among the cerebral palsied is much higher than among normals.

Cerebral palsied children frequently have hearing losses related to their neurological condition, but they are also susceptible to other sources of hearing disorder such as genetic factors, ototoxic medication, and middle ear disease.

More children with athetoid cerebral palsy than those with other types have hearing loss (Table 5.1). However, recent improvement in prenatal and neonatal care of children susceptible to athetosis apparently has reduced its incidence.

THE AUDITORY SYSTEM

It is conventional to divide the hearing mechanism into the peripheral ear and the central auditory system.

Peripheral Ear

The peripheral ear consists of outer, middle, and inner sections. Sound enters through the external auditory meatus of the outer ear. The pinna, by casting an acoustic shadow from back to front, aids in auditory localization, but it is doubtful that it actually collects and directs sound into the ear canal.

In the middle ear, the eardrum transduces acoustic stimuli into vibratory motion which is transmitted to the inner ear via the ossicular chain. The middle ear also matches impedance of outside air and inner ear fluid, and protects against excessively loud sounds by action of the stapedial and tensor tympani muscles.

The inner ear processes vibrations into frequency-related components. Hair cells, resting on the basilar membrane, transduce the vibratory motion into neurological impulses which are transmitted to the brainstem via the VIII nerve. Action of the cochlea is processed further via the olivary-cochlea efferent tract (probably by suppressing some hair cell responses).

TABLE 5.1
Occurrence of Hearing Loss Reported in Several Studies of the Cerebral Palsied

SOURCE	SAMPLE	FINDING*
Byers et al., 1955	19 athetoid	Of 13 cases, 13 testable; 12 with hearing loss
Cunningham & Holt, 1977	athetoids	25% with hearing loss
Fisch, 1957	427 cerebral palsied children in special schools	25% with some hearing loss 16.5% with serious hearing loss
Hattoril, 1966	156 cerebral palsied children	13 with sensorineural (cochlear) hearing loss
Hopkins et al., 1954	summary of several studies	7.2% spastic 22.6% athetoid 13.7% rigidity 18.4% ataxia
Nakano, 1966	318 cerebral palsied children	28% with hearing loss
Rutherford, 1945	49 cerebral palsied children in public school for handicapped	41% with hearing loss more than 15 dB (14% more than 25 dB)
Gerber, 1966	26 day school cerebral palsied pupils	All cerebral palsied children: 59% with hearing loss 50% non-Rh athetoid 100% Rh athetoid 50% spastic
Blakley, 1959	168 with erythroblastosis	17% with sensorineural hearing loss
Pruszewicz et al., 1977	54 extraparamidal cases	52% with hearing loss

*Findings are those reported by each author.

Central Auditory System

The brainstem transmits neurological energy from the cochlea to higher levels. In the brainstem, signals from the two ears are coordinated and auditory neurological energy is processed for acoustic reflexes and for auditory localization.

The cerebral cortex contains the primary sensory area for hearing (Heschl's areas in temporal lobes) and for perception of auditory input (Wernicke's area in the dominant side of the brain). In the cortex, auditory input is integrated with input from the other senses.

Cerebral palsied children may have damage to any of these areas, with symptoms varying according to which part of the auditory system is damaged.

DISORDERS OF THE AUDITORY SYSTEM

Outer and Middle Ear

Diseases of the outer and middle ears produce conductive hearing losses which reduce the loudness of sound reaching the inner ear. Such conditions often are amenable to medical or surgical treatment. For individuals with residual conductive hearing losses after medical or surgical treatment, hearing aids usually are effective.

Inner Ear and VIII Nerve

Sensorineural hearing losses resulting from diseases of the inner ear and VIII nerve present more difficult problems. Usually medical or surgical intervention does not remediate the hearing loss, although it may inhibit progress of the disease.

Sensorineural problems produce loss of acuity, but other problems called *dysacusis*, frequently are present. For example, in cochlear recruitment, the person does not hear low-level sound, but is hypersensitive to higher decibel sounds. If the lesion is in the VIII nerve, fatigue of VIII nerve neurons may cause tone decay which results in fading of the hearing of sounds until there is a period of acoustic rest. Both phenomena (recruitment and tone decay) may contribute to the variable and hard-to-interpret responses of cerebral palsied children. Hearing aids frequently are of benefit for sensorineural problems, but the amount of help is not as great as for conductive hearing losses.

Individuals with sensorineural disease may have vestibular problems resulting in loss of balance. However, these should not be confused with ataxia or movements of the athetoid or spastic child who demonstrates generalized accessory movements, abnormal reflexes, overt signs of cerebral palsy, and speech or language problems. The person with a vestibular problem shows feelings of vertigo, past pointing, abnormal nystigmography results, and lack of typical cerebral palsy signs.

Brainstem

Deficient integration of signals from the peripheral ears by the brainstem results in deficient auditory function such as elevated threshold, deficient localization, confusion when presented with speech signals, difficulty hearing in noise, or lack of auditory summation when fragmentary speech signals are presented differentially to the two ears. Also, the auditory reflexes may be impaired. Damage to the efferent olivary cochlear tract, originating in the brainstem, is suspected to result in less than normal ability to separate auditory signals from noise (Rasmussen & Windle, 1960).

While the reticular formation of the brainstem is not usually considered part of the auditory tract, defects in it may have deleterious auditory effects. The reticular formation is believed to activate or alert the general response system, including responses to acoustic stimuli (Luria, 1973). An affected individual may evidence relatively good auditory threshold acuity if testing is begun at high decibel levels (system alerted), but poor threshold acuity if testing is begun at low levels (system not alerted). Although not well documented, it has been hypothesized that some children with cerebral palsy evidence auditory problems because of reticular formation defects.

Cortex

At the cerebral cortex, hearing dysfunction may be caused by specific brain injury, generalized injury, or malformation. Damage to Heschl's area in either temporal lobe leads to defects in auditory processing such as in auditory localization, perception of rhythm patterns, and confusion when hearing speech. Damage to Wernicke's area leads to auditory aphasia and to other problems.

NORMAL AUDITORY DEVELOPMENT
RELATED TO AUDITORY ASSESSMENT

Neonatal

Shortly after birth it is possible to observe some response to acoustic stimuli, and by 72 hours normal children consistently give eye blink (auropalpebral response), startle (evidenced by general muscular contraction), and change in eye movement (oculogyric response) to soft as well as to loud stimuli (Dedmon & Robinette, 1973). Within a few days there is a change in sucking activity in response to sound (Regan & Charbonneau, 1977), the child appears to be comforted by the mother's voice differentially when compared to voices of other people (Hammond, 1970), and soft voices change the child's behavior—random movements stop and the child appears to be attentive to sound (Ewing & Ewing, 1947).

By 3 months of age, children are comforted by voices, especially the mother's, and continue to exhibit startle responses to sudden and loud sounds (Ewing & Ewing, 1947; Gesell & Armatruda, 1960). Some test procedures for these functions, and the auditory functions normally present at older ages, are given in a later section of this chapter.

Three Months to Twelve Months

At 3 months of age, the child notices familiar sounds (Ewing & Ewing, 1947). By 4 months of age the infant shows a change in heart beat rate in response to sound, probably a precursor to auditory localization (Clifton, 1969), and by 6 months of age the child turns toward familiar sounds. The normal 7-month-old child is readily able to do left-right localizations, but not vertical localization (Ewing & Ewing, 1947; Lowe, 1968).

The child at 12 months usually is able to do front-back localization, and rudimentary vertical localization is apparent. Although the normal child is appreciative of human speech before 12 months of age, responses to speech for audiological assessment are limited during the first year to localization and gaining the child's attention.

Over Twelve Months

At about 12 months of age, the child recognizes some specific words, responds to its name, carries out simple commands, and appears to comprehend simple speech (Ewing & Ewing, 1947).

By 15 to 18 months the child attends to a wide range of sounds and notices them differentially, responds to music by moving rhythmically (Gesell & Armatruda, 1960), and begins to imitate animal sounds and say the names of common animals. By 18 months the child points to body parts upon command. The child now leaves babbling, develops echolalia, and has a wide range of verbal output—although it may not be intelligible. It has vocal inflection and rhythmic patterns which approximate things frequently said in the home.

Usually the normal 3-year-old child can attend to pure tone audiometric tests, without masking, and responds to play audiometry (manipulating a toy in response to tones) (Northern & Downs, 1978). In the normal child, an estimate of hearing status can be obtained from the child's vocal output. This may be absent in the child who has good hearing and intellectual ability, but who lacks motor skills. However, if the child has speech and language appropriate for its chronological age (taking specific motor deficiencies into account), it is a good assumption that a severe hearing loss is not present in the middle range of auditory frequencies.

By 3 years of age the normal child is able to answer questions, follow directions during testing, carry on a conversation, and respond to formal speech reception tests. Typical tasks include asking the child to point to an array of toys or pictures (Newby, 1979; Northern & Downs, 1978; Siegenthaler & Haspiel, 1966). With some children, oral response can be used. Other techniques include following simple directions such as "point to your nose," or "put the doll on the chair." Depending upon previous experiences, the child may keep time with music, sing songs, and in other ways respond to music.

Auditory Maturation

There is an improvement in auditory function throughout infancy and childhood. After age 3, pure tone thresholds improve about 5 decibels, reaching the adult level at about the age of 8 years; speech reception threshold improves by 9 decibels, and speech intelligibility gains approximately 15%. Three-year-old children have about 18 degrees accuracy of auditory localization on the horizontal plane, and reach accuracy of approximately 5 degrees by 8 years of age, with small further improvement through the age of 13 years (Siegenthaler, 1969).

Audiometric standards for pure tones and speech are set for motivated normal young adults at the peak of their auditory functioning. A child's responses should be adjusted for age when making judgments as to functional hearing level, especially if the child is younger than 8 years.

ASSESSMENT OF AUDITORY FUNCTION

Test Rooms

For valid and reliable hearing testing, a special room is needed. A test room has sound-isolating walls, windows, ceiling and floor, and a door with acoustic seals. The interior surfaces are built to reduce sound reflections. Principles of selecting a commercially built test room have been described (Siegenthaler, 1982).

The room is served by a combined pure tone and speech audiometer, with the audiologist seated outside the viewing window and the subject within the room. For many cerebral palsied children it is better to have the audiologist use a portable audiometer in the room with the child. This provides for more immediate contact and control with the child, which may be necessary. Because usually live voice is used with difficult-to-test subjects, speech audiometry requires external placement of the audiologist and audiometer while the earphones and loudspeakers remain in the test room.

Hearing Tests

The audiologist's armamentarium contains many tests and procedures, not all equally useful in the evaluation of cerebral palsied children.

Pure Tone Audiogram. The pure tone audiogram charts the subject's hearing level by frequency for the ears individually at octave frequencies. This is done by air conduction (under an earphone), and by bone conduction using an oscillator, usually on the mastoid process. If acuity of the two ears is noticeably different, masking noise is applied in the better ear while testing the poorer one, but the use of masking is difficult with young children or those with CNS problems. Information gained from the audiogram is significant for indicating the decibel level of hearing acuity, pattern of audiogram, and site of lesion.

Testing with pure tones from a loudspeaker is inaccurate because of difficulty in establishing a sound field without significant standing waves. However, sometimes it is the only pure tone technique possible with a child.

Many cerebral palsied children have relatively good hearing in the low frequencies and rapid drop-off in the middle and high frequencies. Because the important frequencies for understanding speech are the middle frequencies of 500 Hz, 1000 Hz, and 2000 Hz, it is common practice to obtain the mean decibel threshold value for these three tones in an ear, although some audiologists prefer to use the two best across the three frequencies. Either method gives an overall estimate of hearing acuity and an estimate of the speech reception threshold if it cannot be tested directly. The high frequencies, 4000 Hz and above, contribute much less to speech intelligibility, even to so-called high frequency speech sounds such as sibilants.

Bone conduction threshold testing is intended to measure the sensitivity of the inner ear. If bone conduction is good while air conduction acuity is significantly reduced (air-bone gap), there is an obstructive or conductive deafness in the outer or middle ear. This is seen in children with impacted ear wax, middle ear problems such as otitis media, or microtic ear. If bone conduction is reduced and essentially equal to air conduction which also is reduced (no air-bone gap), there is an inner ear or VIII nerve lesion (sensorineural problem). Air conduction thresholds, which show a markedly greater loss for high than for low frequencies, are also associated with sensorineural hearing losses.

Audiologists may not test all frequencies, or may test down to 15 or 25 decibels rather than seek thresholds. Adequate hearing for the development of speech often can be demonstrated even though a threshold audiogram is not obtained. If only limited testing can be done, the frequency of choice should be 1000 Hz because its threshold correlates best with speech reception.

Speech Audiometry

Speech Reception Threshold.   The ability to hear speech is measured in part by the speech reception threshold (SRT), the lowest decibel level where speech can be understood 50% of the time. It may be called word threshold (WT) if words are used for testing or spondee threshold (ST) if spondee words are used. The words may be represented by pictures to which the subject points, a technique usable with cerebral palsied children who have no intelligible speech. Those who do not have manual ability may use a head pointer, turn the head, or cast the eyes to a picture. Speech reception threshold has a high correlation with audiometric average (Siegenthaler & Strand, 1964).

An SRT should include a notation about the speech material used because the exact test procedures are important factors, especially when evaluating children with cerebral palsy for whom adaptations or special tests are needed.

Speech Intelligibility.   This perhaps is of even greater significance than speech reception threshold. Testing involves the use of a list of words given at a constant decibel level, such as the usual loudness of conversation. The subject identifies each word, and a percent correct score is obtained.

Speech Intelligibility (SI), sometimes noted as Word Recognition Score (WRS), is measured by having the subject repeat the test word as each is given over an earphone or loudspeaker. A Speech Discrimination (SD) or Word Discrimination Score (WDS) employs a small, closed set of items. The subject is asked either to report *same* or *different* if a pair of items is presented, or to indicate which item is said (as when a set of words is available and only one word is called).

PB Max refers to the best speech intelligibility test score the subject can attain under optimum conditions in a quiet test room and the highest loudness level which the subject will accept without introducing distortion, recruitment, or tolerance problems. The usual practice is to use phonetically balanced (PB) word lists; hence the notation PB Max. Other word lists may be used to obtain a maximum score.

For assessing a subject's daily living function a discrimination, intelligibility, or recognition score at the decibel level of normal conversational speech is obtained. This is usually at 40 dB above the normal speech threshold. In this case, the 40 dB should be noted as 40 dB HL (Hearing Level) because it is referenced to normals.

To obtain PB Max or an equivalent, however, requires a stimulus level at least 40 dB above the specific subject's SRT. In this case, the stimuli are at 40 dB SL (Sensation Level). The reference here is the individual's threshold. Unfortunately, some audiologists indicate a test score, but not whether it was for maximum or for normal conversational speech. If not specified, it is most likely a PB Max score. It is wise to check the level at which a given word intelligibility score was obtained so the score can be interpreted correctly.

Alternate forms of intelligibility testing have been developed using pictures. The child selects the correct word from a closed set of pictures, and the test score is then corrected for chance.

Because speech intelligibility is related to the person's everyday understanding of speech, the higher the percentage the better. However, a direct conversion from test score to percentage understanding of speech is not made because many other factors are related to speech understanding in daily living.

If standard practice is followed, neither a speech reception threshold nor speech intelligibility score is obtained while the subject can view the audiologist's face. Perhaps a better estimate of functional ability to understand speech is to repeat the tests while the subject watches the speaker's lips. This produces a combined look-and-listen test result which is closer to the normal situation than is testing without lipreading.

Unfortunately, whisper, voice, and noise tests have limited possibilities to assess frequency characteristics of a child's hearing, although they are useful for assessing the gross level of hearing. They have low frequency as well as middle and high frequency components. A response is obtained if the subject hears only one of the components.

Speech Detection Threshold (SDT or SD). This threshold may be noted for a subject with whom a standard SRT cannot be obtained. In persons with uncomplicated peripheral hearing loss, the SDT is about 10 decibels lower than the SRT. However, one cannot assume that if a child with cerebral palsy gives an SDT, the SRT is 10 decibels above that level. Many auditory or nonauditory factors may be responsible for failure to understand speech.

Localization

Auditory localization requires two good peripheral ears, and is mediated by the brainstem and the primary sensory auditory cortex (Heschl's areas on the temporal lobes). Cerebral palsied children who do not localize may be suspected of having unilateral hearing loss, severe bilateral hearing loss, or CNS damage.

Additionally, many cerebral palsied children make significantly poorer auditory-visual associations than normals, and their auditory localization dysfunction may be due to this inability (Birch & Belmont, 1965). In other cerebral palsied children with head tilt, body tilt, constant head motion, or lack of head control, localization is deficient because the child is unable to locate a sound spatially, and because the child lacks the habituation experiences necessary to develop auditory localization.

Audiology does not have standardized tests for measuring auditory localization, but audiologists improvise procedures to estimate this ability. One procedure is to call from loudspeakers at different positions in the test room. Another is to place the child in the middle of a room, eyes closed, while the audiologist calls or makes noises from different positions. Often teachers, therapists, or child care workers can report a child's localization for naturally occurring sounds in the environment.

Other Areas.   Other auditory functions include figure-background perception, synthesis of fragmented speech signals into meaningful words or phrases, reaction time to sound, and central auditory perception. None of these currently is measured using well established standardized procedures, although several tests are available for central auditory perception (Katz, 1978).

Central auditory function tests are demanding, and they require good subject cooperation and understanding. Lack of motor skills, short attention span, and poor speech ability are problems in younger cerebral palsied children that limit validity of formal tests. Tests for central auditory perception may include speech discrimination in noise, staggered spondee words, accelerated speech, filtered speech, binaural integration, and auditory sequencing. Given a sophisticated staff who are able to spend time with a cerebral palsied child, observations can be accrued informally which often provide the information gained from formal tests in these areas.

Visual figure-background differentiation has been well documented among brain-damaged children (Cruickshank, et al., 1965) but auditory figure-background perception has been researched relatively little. Brain-injured children do more poorly on auditory discrimination in noise than normals due to cortical lesions, rather than general or specific auditory factors (Schlanger, 1958).

Cerebral palsied children, as a group, have poorer than normal auditory figure-background differentiation in noise, but there are wide variations among individuals. Visual figure-background varies independently from auditory figure-background perception, contrary to the view that figure-background perception is a general factor rather than a specific factor for each sense modality (Goldstein, 1965; Proctor, 1968; Ross, 1960).

Deficiency in the efferent auditory tract from olivary nucleus to cochlea may account for the auditory figure-background problem in cerebral palsied children. This pathway is said to enhance the signal-to-noise ratio or conversely, to provide a poor signal-to-noise ratio when damaged. Poor signal-to-noise ratio probably is related to hyperactivity, distractability, and other poor performances by brain-injured children, including the cerebral palsied (Protti, 1983).

SPECIAL PROCEDURES

Operant Conditioning Testing

For individuals difficult to test by ordinary audiometry, operant conditioning techniques may be used. Usually the procedure calls for obtaining pure tone thresholds, although it can be adapted for other stimuli. Conditioning is obtained by rewarding the child for a stimulus-response event, but not rewarding (or even punishing) the child for a response-no-stimulus event. It may be necessary to work through a training period of stimulus-unconditioned response leading to stimulus-conditioned response, or it may be sufficient to explain or demonstrate what is desired behavior.

An early version of this type of test was the Peep Show (Dix & Halpike, 1947). The child pressed a button to light a doll house and see a rewarding scene. Other versions include rewarding the child with a slide show or a moving toy (Kaplan & Siegenthaler, 1958; Green, 1958). Such procedures facilitate testing difficult-to-test children, give thresholds in good agreement with other procedures, and obtain more complete testing than other techniques. An adaptation is to arrange a box with a hinged cover and a micro-switch. A cerebral palsied child who has only gross movements can use the whole hand, an elbow, a head wand or a foot movement to operate the switch. Interlocking the switch with a tone-on switch is useful, but not necessary.

More formalized operant conditioning techniques with associated electrical and mechanical equipment have been used with many types of handicapped children, although most evaluations were with the mentally retarded. Specific conditioning protocols, reinforcement schedules, and types of rewards and punishments have been described (Fulton & Spradlin, 1969). For the physically handicapped child, adaptations of the response mode, ability to be conditioned, allowance for slow response times, and appropriateness of reward are significant considerations. Considerable training time with the equipment may be necessary for success using this technique.

Behavior Observation

In a sense, behavioral observation is the simplest hearing testing method; if someone notices that a cerebral palsied child does not seem to respond to environmental sound or voice, a behavior observation test has been made. The Ewings (1947) described the hearing assessment of children using many behavioral observation techniques. Behavior observation relies on naturally occurring environmental sounds, tester-initiated sounds, and human voice. Because such stimuli can be specified only grossly for frequency and sound level, and they nearly always contain a wide frequency spectrum, eventually more exacting and formal audiometric study is desirable. Even so, behavior observation techniques compare favorably with follow-up audiometry (Lowe, 1968; Shimakura, 1976).

For many cerebral palsied children, behavioral observation may be the only approach possible. This procedure can be formalized somewhat by combining it with a speech audiometer reading made in a hearing test room to allow decibel level specification, at least for the most intense component of the stimulus sound.

A well-developed protocol for behavioral observation testing was presented by Bendet (1976) as a checklist of responses to sounds related to child developmental levels.

Physiological Tests

An audiological procedure which once enjoyed popularity is the psychogalvanic skin response (PGSR) test, also known as galvanic skin response (GSR) or electrodermal response (EDR) (Hardy & Pauls, 1952). The procedure involves observation of the conditioned response of the sympathetic nervous system (sweating of the palms) to tones. Experimental results with children having cerebral palsy were mixed; the technique did not yield valid and reliable results on 22 of 30 subjects, forty percent of handicapped subjects could not be conditioned (Lehrhoff, 1961; Koch, 1965), and GSR testing was not successful with children who could not be tested by other standard methods (O'Neill, Oyer, & Hillis, 1961).

A recent development is aural impedance testing. Its most useful aspect is the tympanogram, which charts eardrum mobility as a function of air pressure in the external ear canal. It is a major tool for the detection of middle ear conditions and has been successful with some cerebral palsied children (Keith, Murphy, & Martin, 1976). Many cerebral palsied children, however, have involuntary movements which make it difficult to mount the impedance audiometry equipment on their heads or to obtain an adequate ear canal seal when the test probe is inserted. Some of the newer equipment which is hand-held, self-contained, and automatic should increase the application of impedance audiometry to cerebral palsied children.

Another recent development is cortical (EEG) and brainstem evoked response (BSER) audiometry. The general principle here is that as neurological responses to auditory stimuli (clicks or tone bursts) are transmitted through the brainstem to the cerebral cortex, surface electrodes detect the electrical activity of the nervous system. Results are processed by an averaging computer to enhance the response display.

Use of this technique with handicapped children has had mixed success, but cortical response audiometry was found to be useful for children with cerebral palsy (Bagley, 1971; Mathis & Graf, 1974). Apparently the procedure presented no significant testing problems, despite a longer latency of response. It often was necessary, however, to use sedation with cerebral palsied children.

Some cerebral palsied children demonstrate auditory cortical responses to sounds 30 decibels or less while asleep, yet appear to be severely deaf when awake. They lack speech output, understand little speech by listening, and attempt lip-reading to understand what is said to them. Other cerebral palsied children with speech have similar asleep and awake test results (Taylor, 1962). This suggests that some cerebral palsied children are inhibited in auditory behavior when awake, even though they have adequate peripheral ears. Perhaps they lack ability to process the mass of sensory information to which they are subjected when awake. Such inability can explain lack of response, variability of response to sound, and limitations of hearing aids for some children with cerebral palsy.

Tonic head and neck positions adversely influence obtaining electrical responses, making this procedure inappropriate for cerebral palsied children who cannot maintain a relaxed supine or prone position (Habafellner & Muller, 1976). While the EEG test appears to be useful for many children, it serves as an additional rather than a definitive test in the auditory evaluation of children difficult to test. Apparently only 37% give readable responses, and interpretation of responses related to functional hearing is difficult (Biesalski, Leightner, & Muller-Gerhard, 1976).

The large body of research which would support the use of these procedures for standard clinical practice remains to be done. The current status of evoked response audiometry was summarized by Protti (1983) who indicated that: (a) such testing may not be sensitive to all brainstem involvements even though positive findings have site-of-lesion implications; (b) negative findings do not rule out central auditory processing dysfunction because brainstem stimulus-response is nonspeech in nature and a poor indicator of central auditory dysfunction; and (c) there is not a strong relationship between abnormal performance on subjective tests of brainstem function and BSER.

AUDIOGRAM INTERPRETATION

Decibel Level

It is common practice to use the average audiometric air conduction threshold across the middle three frequencies to classify the level of hearing acuity. Table 5.2 gives approximate average decibel hearing levels, descriptive terms, and implications for children whose hearing losses are

TABLE 5.2
Decibel Levels of Hearing Acuity, Descriptive Terms, and Some Implications

dB LEVEL*	DESCRIPTOR FOR HEARING LEVEL	IMPLICATIONS IF NOT REMEDIATED
15 dB	Normal	If speech discrimination and other hearing functions are normal, no auditory follow-up.
15–25 dB	Borderline (sometimes included in normal category)	May have difficulty hearing low level sounds; hearing adequate for speech and language development; hearing aid use only occasionally, possibly for alerting.
25–40 dB	Mild	Difficulty hearing speech; often results in speech (articulation) defects for the less intense speech sounds; language essentially normal; mild gain hearing aid necessary for adequate normal functioning.
40–60 dB	Moderate	Considerable difficulty hearing speech; speech and language development not normal; hearing aid beneficial.
60–80 dB	Severe	Can hear only fragments of normal speech; speech and oral language grossly defective or absent; voice affected; hearing aid beneficial; 60 dB or worse used as legal definition of *educationally deaf* in some contexts.
Worse than 80 dB	Profound	Little ability to hear speech; speech and oral language grossly defective or absent; often rely on manual or other non-oral communication; hearing aid may be beneficial; are *educationally deaf*.

*Based on PTA and/or SRT.

uncorrected or uncompensated. For children with cerebral palsy, the implications for each level of hearing acuity are more depressed because of their neuromuscular condition, learning problems, sensory or perceptual problems, and associated medical or health problems. For example, a child with severe oral-motor problems but with good hearing may have to rely on nonoral communication because of speech inability.

Hearing level (HL) compares an individual's acuity with that of the normal hearing population, and is seen on the air conduction audiogram as decibel threshold deviation from audiometric 0 dB. This may be adjusted for age of the child, but notation of age correction should be made to avoid confusion.

Hearing loss also uses audiometric thresholds, but indicates how much an individual's hearing acuity has changed over time. If a child had an initial hearing threshold of 10 decibels, but it changed later to 45 decibels, there would be a 35 decibel hearing loss. Often hearing loss and hearing level are used interchangeably, but incorrectly.

Shape of Audiogram

If an audiogram shows about equal acuity across frequencies, the mean threshold level is a good indication of overall hearing level. However, if the audiogram shows good hearing in the low frequencies with poorer hearing in the middle and high frequencies, a relatively good threshold average but relatively poor speech discrimination may result. Also factors of dysacusis such as recruitment, tone decay, and auditory aphasia—which are not revealed by a threshold audiogram—may place limitations on the functional use of a cerebral palsied child's hearing.

Considerations in Testing the Cerebral Palsied Child

While knowing the site of lesion, the etiology, and the classification of a cerebral palsied child's condition may be of help in planning programs, there is danger of stereotyping or having incorrect expectations of the child. One should consider the hearing of the child as revealed by physical examination and, in the present context, by formal audiological evaluation. Minimal cues to hearing should be observed, but the careful audiologist will rely on overt behaviors, taking into account physical limitations of the child. Not to do so leads to unrealistic assessment of the child.

Objective audiometry (e.g., brainstem or cortical responses) too often is even more subjective than the usual test procedures. It gives information about the operation of the child's CNS, but less regarding the child's perceptual processes or auditory associations. Standard audiological practice continues to rely on subjective audiometry, with objective techniques for confirmation or backup.

In all procedures for the difficult-to-test child, multiple observations with various stimuli having known sound levels are necessary. The audiologist must be careful to separate responses to test stimuli from spontaneously occurring activity. However, assume a stimulus is presented a number of times without response, but then a response is observed. How should it be scored? If it can be determined that the response was related to the stimulus, that response should be given full credit.

It is appropriate to begin at a level of testing just below the child's best level of participation. To begin at a too easy level uses up the child's reservoir of responses before his or her level of competence is reached. Conversely, it is prudent to assure some early successful test performance before moving to more demanding tasks for the child. To begin at too demanding a level runs the risk of discouraging or confusing the child.

Sometimes it is difficult to keep in mind, when the audiologist has available a wide range of sophisticated and exacting tests of hearing function, just what the goal should be. The goal is not to complete successfully a specific test procedure nor to make measurements on a pair of ears. The goal is to assess the auditory function of the cerebral palsied child, especially in terms of implications for that child's maximum life adjustment.

It is not within the scope of the present chapter to discuss extensively the remedial or training procedures for cerebral palsied children with hearing handicaps. In general, procedures for the hearing stimulation of these children are very similar to those for the deaf and for the learning disabled child, especially regarding acoustic stimulation (see Bess & McConnell, 1981; Ewing & Ewing, 1947; Newby & Papelka, 1985; Saunders, 1982).

In this context, the cerebral palsied child would not be of specific interest. Rather, the focus here is on the child's hearing problem, which requires essentially the same audiological training procedures as for other children with auditory dysfunction. Modifications to adapt to the physical needs of the child are important and necessary, but the goal of auditory development and ways to facilitate that are related to generalized principles for bringing about auditory development in all children.

REFERENCES

Bagley, H. (1971). Present day scope and limitations of evoked response audiometry. *Review of Laryngology, Otology and Rhinology, 92*, 753–763.

Bendet, R. (1976). Evaluating hearing of the low-developmental level child. *Asha, 18*, 407–414.

Bess, F., & McConnell, F. (Eds.) (1981). *Audiology, education, and the hearing impaired child.* St. Louis, MO: C. V. Mosby.

Biesalski, P., Leightner, H., & Muller-Gerhard, N. (1976). Relations between electric response audiometry, conventional audiometry and psychodiagnostic examination in hearing impaired children. *Audiology, 15*, 376–383.

Birch, H., & Belmont, L. (1965). Auditory-visual integration in brain-damaged and normal children. *Developmental Medicine and Child Neurology, 7*, 135–144.

Blakley, R. (1959). Erythroblastosis and perceptive hearing loss. *Journal of Speech and Hearing Research, 2*, 5–13.

Byers, R., Paine, R., & Crothers, B. (1955). Extrapyramidal cerebral palsy with hearing loss following erythroblastosis. *Pediatrics, 15*, 248–254.

Clifton, R. (1969). The heart rate response of four-month-old infants to auditory stimuli. *Journal of Exceptional Child Psychology, 7*, 122–135.

Cruickshank, W. M., Bice, H. V., Wallen, N. E., & Lynch, K. (1965). *Perception and cerebral palsy* (2nd ed.). Syracuse, NY: Syracuse University Press.

Cunningham, C., & Holt, K. (1977). Problems in diagnosis and management of children with cerebral palsy and deafness. *Developmental Medicine and Child Neurology, 19*, 479–484.

Dedmon, D., & Robinette, M. (1973). The acoustic reflex as a tool for neonatal screening. *Audicebel, 22*, 202–210.

Dix, M. & Halpike, C. (1947). The peep show: new techniques for pure tone audiometry in children. *British Medical Journal, 2*, 7–19.

Ewing, I., & Ewing, A. (1947). *Opportunity and the deaf child*. London: University of London Press.

Fisch, L. (1957, December). Hearing impairment and cerebral palsy. *Speech, 21*.

Fulton, R., & Spradlin, J. (1969). Conditioning and audiologic assessment. In R. Fulton & L. Lloyd (Eds.), *Auditory assessment of the difficult to test* (pp. 154–178). Baltimore, MD: Williams and Wilkins.

Gerber, S. (1966). Cerebral palsy and hearing loss. *Cerebral Palsy Journal, 27*, 6–7.

Gesell, A., & Armatruda, C. (1960). *Developmental diagnosis: Normal and abnormal child development*. New York: Paul B. Holber.

Goldstein, J. (1965). *Auditory and visual figure-background perception in adult aphasics*. Unpublished master's thesis, The Pennsylvania State University, PA.

Green, D. (1958). The peep-show: A simple inexpensive modification of the peepshow. *Journal of Speech and Hearing Disorders, 23*, 118–120.

Habafellner, H., & Muller, G. (1976). Sequelae of head and neck positions on auditory performance. *Neuropaediatrie, 7*, 273–278.

Hammond, J. (1970). Hearing and response in the newborn. *Developmental Medicine and Child Neurology, 12*, 1.

Hardy, W., & Pauls, M. (1952). The test situation in PGSR audiometry. *Journal of Speech and Hearing Disorders, 17*, 13–24.

Hattoril, H. (1966). Hearing impairment in cerebral palsy. *Practice of Otology, 59*, 648–653.

Hopkins, T., Bice, H., & Cotton, M. (1954). *Evaluation and education of the cerebral palsied child*. Washington, DC: International Council for Exceptional Children.

Kaplan, H., & Siegenthaler, B. (1958). A comparison of picture response and hand raising technique in pure tone audiometry with young children. *Laryngoscope, 65*, 548–557.

Katz, J. (1978). Evaluation of central dysfunction. In J. Katz (Ed.), *Handbook of Clinical Audiology* (2nd ed.) (pp. 233–243). Baltimore, MD: Williams and Wilkins.

Keith, R., Murphy, K., & Martin, F. (1976). Acoustic reflex measurements in children with cerebral palsy. *Folia Phoniatrica, 28*, 311–314.

Koch, A. (1956). *A comparative study of auditory thresholds of spastic cerebral palsied adults and non-handicapped adults as measured by standard audiometric and psychogalvanic skin resistance procedures*. Unpublished doctoral dissertation, Boston University, MA.

Lehrhoff, I. (1961). A study of PGSR testing of Rh athetoids. *Annals of Otology, Rhinology, and Laryngology, 70*, 234–238.

Lowe, A. (1968). Audiological measures in the early care of cerebral palsied children. *Neue Blaetter fuer Taubstummenbildung, 22,* 317–322.

Luria, A. (1973). *The working brain: An introduction to neuropsychology.* New York: Basic Books.

Mathis, A., & Graf, K. (1974). Evoked response audiometry in children with cerebral palsy. *Archiv fuer Ohren-Nasen-und Kehlkopfheilkunde, 203,* 261–281.

Nakano, T. (1966). Research hearing impairment in cerebral infantile palsied school children. *International Audiology, 5,* 159–161.

Newby, H. (1979). *Audiology* (4th ed.). Englewood Cliffs, NJ: Prentice-Hall.

Newby, H., & Papelka, G. (1985). *Audiology* (5th ed.). Englewood Cliffs, NJ: Prentice-Hall.

Northern, J., & Downs, M. (1978). *Hearing in children* (2nd ed.). Baltimore, MD: Williams & Wilkins.

O'Neill, J., Oyer, J., & Hillis, J. (1961). Audiometric procedures used with children. *Journal of Speech and Hearing Disorders, 26,* 61–66.

Proctor, A. (1968). *Auditory and visual figure-background perception in athetoid cerebral palsied children.* Unpublished master's thesis, The Pennsylvania State University, University Park, PA.

Protti, E. (1983). Brainstem auditory pathways and auditory processing disorders: Diagnostic implications of subjective and objective tests. In E. Lasky & J. Katz (Eds.), *Central auditory processing disorders* (pp. 117–140). Austin, TX: PRO-ED.

Pruszewicz, A., Obrebowski, A., & Fgorzalewicz, B. (1977). Selected problems in the hearing, voice, and speech disturbances in the extrapyramidal form of cerebral palsy. *Folia Phoniatrica, 29,* 302–310.

Rasmussen, G., & Windle, W. (Eds.). (1960). *Neuromechanism of the auditory and vestibular systems.* Springfield, IL: Charles C Thomas.

Regan, J., & Charbonneau, M. (1977). Sound response to sucking patterns in infants. *Audiological and Hearing Education, 3,* 6–10.

Ross, F. (1960). *Auditory figure-background relationships for speech hearing in cerebral palsied and normal subjects.* Unpublished master's thesis, The Pennsylvania State University, University Park, PA.

Rutherford, B. (1945). Hearing loss in cerebral palsied children. *Journal of Speech Disorders, 10,* 237–240.

Saunders, D. (1982). *Aural rehabilitation* (2nd ed.). Englewood Cliffs, NJ: Prentice-Hall.

Schlanger, B. (1958). Results of varying presentations to brain injured children of an auditory word discrimination test. *American Journal of Mental Deficiency, 63,* 464–468.

Shimakura, Y. (1976). Audiometry for a severely retarded infant. *Bulletin of the Tokyo Metropolitan Rehabilitation Center for Physical and Mental Handicaps, 2,* 1–7.

Siegenthaler, B. (1969). Maturation of auditory abilities in children. *International Audiology, 7,* 59–71.

Siegenthaler, B. (1982). Forum: A primer of hearing test room considerations. *Volta Review, 84,* 285–290.

Siegenthaler, B., & Haspiel, G. (1966). *Development of two standardized measures of hearing for speech by children.* USOE Cooperative Research Program. (Project No. 2372).

Siegenthaler, B., & Strand, B. (1964). Audiogram average methods and SRT scores. *Journal of the Acoustical Society of America, 36,* 389–393.

Taylor, I. (1962). Diagnosis of deafness in cerebral palsy. *Spastic Quarterly, 11,* 37–50.

CHAPTER 6

Visual Problems

Robert H. Duckman

Duckman points out that persons with cerebral palsy might have any of the visual problems found in the general population and, in addition, they are at risk for ocular-motor dysfunction and visual perceptual disorders. Understanding of these problems and their far-reaching effect on learning and performance is important for all disciplines involved in rehabilitation.

1. *Trace the path of a visual stimulus from its entry into the eye to its activation of the visual cortex of the occipital lobe, describing the structures through which the stimulus passes and how the stimulus is affected by each structure.*

2. *Inability of the eyes to maintain visual alignment is found in a high percentage of cerebral palsied children. What are the manifestations of this condition and how is it treated?*

3. *For each of the following aspects of the visual process describe (a) normal function and how it develops, and (b) aberrant function as it might be seen in cerebral palsy:* acuity, fixation, tracking, vergence, refraction, accommodation, fusion, *and* phoria.

4. *Why are children with severe motor handicaps at risk for visual perception dysfunction?*

5. *With several nonhandicapped children, practice each of the training activities described by Duckman.*

INTRODUCTION

The total visual process involves *input* from the eye, *processing* of the input by the central nervous system, and *output* which reveals how the individual interprets and uses the visual input. Persons with cerebral palsy are at risk for difficulties with all parts of the visual process. When present, visual problems interfere with education and with progress in therapies. It is important that parents, teachers, and therapists be aware of any visual problems and that appropriate steps be taken to remediate them.

THE HUMAN VISUAL SYSTEM

The following brief description of the visual system will prepare the readers for later discussions of visual problems in cerebral palsy. Mueller and Rudolph (1970) and Wertenbaker (1981) provide more comprehensive, yet simply written, descriptions.

Light enters the eye through the cornea, then passes through the aqueous humor, the pupil, the crystalline lens and the vitreous humor to come to focus on an area of the retina called the fovea (Figure 6.1). In the light receptor cells of the retina, light is changed to neural impulses which are transmitted via the optic nerve to the thalamus and from there to visual areas in the occipital lobe. Some fibers pass from the thalamus to the midbrain. The right half of each eye is connected with the right visual cortex and the left halves connect with the left visual cortex.

Light rays are refracted (bent) by the cornea and the crystalline lens. Thickness of the crystalline lens, which determines the amount of refraction, is varied by action of the ciliary muscle. Another muscle, the iris, dilates or constricts the pupil in response to light conditions. Movements of each eye are produced by six extrinsic muscles. Normally, the extrinsic muscles of the two eyes act together so both eyes will receive the same image.

Visual Acuity

Visual acuity may be defined as the smallest object whose form can be identified. Many procedures for measurement of visual acuity have been developed.

Snellen Chart. The Snellen Chart consists of rows of letters which progressively decrease in size. Visual acuity is expressed by a fraction which compares the person being tested with "normal" vision. For example, a person who at 20 feet can barely read letters of the same size a normal person can barely read would be said to have 20/20 or normal visual acuity. A person with visual acuity of 20/200 would be able to see at 20 feet what a person with normal acuity would see at 200 feet.

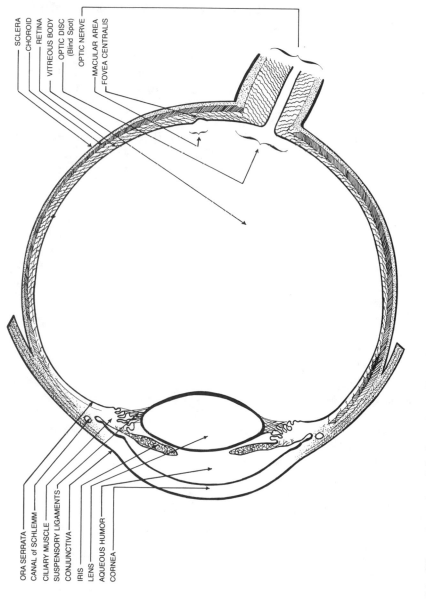

SCLERA
CHOROID
RETINA
VITREOUS BODY
OPTIC DISC
(Blind Spot)
OPTIC NERVE

MACULAR AREA
FOVEA CENTRALIS

ORA SERRATA
CANAL of SCHLEMM
CILIARY MUSCLE
SUSPENSORY LIGAMENTS
CONJUNCTIVA
IRIS
LENS
AQUEOUS HUMOR
CORNEA

Figure 6.1. Schematic section of the human eye. (Reproduced with permission of the American Optometric Association.)

Visually Evoked Potentials (VEPs). Electrodes are placed on the scalp in the area of the occipital cortex and electrophysiological measurements are taken as the patient watches flashing checkerboard patterns which are gradually reduced in size until no electrophysiological activity is observed. The checkerboard size, at this point, may be converted to a visual acuity value.

Optokinetic Nystagmus (OKN). Black and white stripes moving across a patient's visual field will evoke an involuntary oscillation of the eyes. If the stripes are gradually reduced in width, the point where OKN disappears is where the eyes can no longer resolve the black and white stripes as separate entities. This can be converted to a visual acuity measurement if the test distance and the width of the stripes is known.

Forced Preferential Looking (FPL). It is well-established that infants prefer to look at patterned fields over unpatterned fields (Fantz, 1958). The FPL procedure makes use of this behavior by presenting a homogenous field and a striped field simultaneously. An unbiased observer, watching the child's eye movements, decides which side the child prefers. As the stripes get narrower and fall below the infant's ability to resolve the pattern, then there is no preference, since both fields appear homogenous (Teller, 1979). Although the procedure loses its effectiveness in a normal population at about the age of 10 months, it can be extended in a neurologically impaired population up to at least 4 years (Duckman & Selenow, 1983).

Blindness

Legal Blindness. Each of the states has its own definition of legal blindness. Generally, it is defined as best *corrected* visual acuity of 20/200 or less in the *better* eye, or a visual field of 20 degrees or less. Visual field refers to the area or extent of physical space visible to an eye in a given position (usually referred to as peripheral or side vision). A person's normal visual field, while looking straight ahead, is approximately 65 degrees inward and 95 degrees outward (Schapero, Cline, & Hofstetter, 1968). Therefore it is possible to be categorized legally blind with 20/20 visual acuity if there is a significant visual field loss.

Functional Blindness. Each individual has specific visual needs which require specific visual function. When a person is not able to perform a given task due to decrement in vision, that person is said to be functionally blind. Functional blindness is task specific and different for each person. For example, if a person has 20/400 visual acuity (best corrected), but only needs to ambulate about the house, the chances are that that person will be able to function within the environment with the decreased vision. However, if the same individual needs to drive a car, that person is functionally blind for the task of driving.

Cortical Blindness.   It is possible to have a total loss of vision in all or part of the visual field due to a lesion in the striate cortex while all subcortical functions remain intact. Cortical blindness, sometimes referred to as "mind blindness," is characterized by the patient's lack of subjective awareness of the disability.

Ocular Motility

Abnormal Muscle Function.   Normally the six extraocular muscles (EOMs) of the right and the left eyes work together to produce coordinated eye movements. Paralysis or paresis of any of these muscles may limit eye movement in the direction controlled by the affected muscle, or it may cause an inability of the eyes to maintain visual alignment, a condition referred to as strabismus. Esotropia is an inward strabismus (crossed-eyes), exotropia is an outward strabismus (wall-eyed), and hyper- (upward) or hypo- (downward) tropia is a vertical disalignment of the eyes. In strabismus, which may be constant or intermittent, one eye fixates while the other eye turns. If the fixation alternates between eyes, it is referred to as an alternating strabismus. Nystagmus, an involuntary oscillation of the eyes, is an expression of some disorder of the visual, neurological, or vestibular mechanisms. It is frequently congenital in nature, and difficult to correct (Davidson, 1974). Biofeedback has been used with some success to slow down nystagmoid movement in motivated and intelligent patients.

Ocular-Motor Skills.   Normal eyes perform a variety of motor acts which are essential for effective visual function.

Fixation.   Maintaining one or both foveas directed at an object of regard requires a delicate balance of equal and opposite stimulation to antagonistic EOMs of the same eye (under monocular viewing) and an even more delicate balance under binocular conditions.

Pursuit Eye Movements.   To maintain the image of a moving object on the fovea, the speed and direction of the eye movements must match the speed and direction of the target. These movements are also referred to as tracking movements.

Saccadic Eye Movements.   Transfer of gaze from one fixation point to another is accomplished by a rapid movement which is called a saccadic movement, (e.g., at the end of a line of text, the eyes saccade to the beginning of the next line). Because the movement is rapid, vision is blurred while the eyes are moving.

Convergence and Divergence.   Usually when the eyes track or saccade, both eyes move simultaneously in the same direction; however, when converging to fixate at near point, or diverging when shifting gaze from near to far, the eyes move in opposite directions. Movements of the two eyes in the same direction are called conjunctive movements (saccades and pursuits); those in the opposite direction are called dysjunctive movements (convergence and divergence).

Refraction

Refraction is the bending of light rays as they pass from one medium to another. A straight stick partially immersed in water appears to bend from the point where it enters the water. Light rays passing through a prism deviate to a new direction. In the eye, the cornea and crystalline lens refract light. Refractive power is measured in diopters. The normal eye has approximately 60 diopters of refractive power, which is the amount needed to bend light entering the eye to focus on the retina.

Refractive Errors. Inappropriate bending may prevent light rays from coming to a focus on the retina. Too much refraction, as in *myopia* (nearsightedness), focuses the image in front of the retina resulting in blurring distance vision. In *hyperopia* (farsightedness), the light rays do not come to focus by the time they reach the retina. In *astigmatism*, irregularity in the curvature of the cornea causes the light rays to be bent different amounts as they pass through different dimensions of the cornea. Lenses, commonly called "glasses" are used to correct refractive errors. For myopia, concave, or minus, lenses decrease the amount of refraction; for hyperopia, convex, or plus, lenses increase the amount of refraction. Lenses for astigmatism are more complex since they must correct for the irregularities of the cornea.

Accommodation

To produce clear vision at near, as for reading, the eye must increase its refractive power by action of the ciliary muscle to change the curvature of the crystalline lens, a process called accommodation. In young eyes, large changes in lens curvature are possible because the consistency of the lens material is soft. With aging, the lens substance gradually becomes harder. Once the lens is too hard to change shape easily, reading glasses are needed to provide refractive power which the crystalline lens can no longer produce.

Close work such as reading and writing requires simultaneous convergence and accommodation. By action of an "associated reflex," accommodation is accompanied by convergence and vice versa. This creates a situation where the hyperope without glasses must accommodate to see clearly, but since this accommodation is reflexively accompanied by convergence, which is not needed for distance viewing, strabismus may result. This is referred to as an accommodative esotropia (i.e., the esotropia is a result of the convergence induced by the accommodation necessary to make distance vision clear to the hyperope). Often this kind of strabismus will be greatly reduced just by applying convex lenses to relax the accommodation.

Fusion

Under binocular conditions each eye receives visual input, and each eye independently relays information to the brain. Yet we usually see a single image because the retinal points stimulated by light are projected to corresponding points in the brain where the two inputs are fused into a single perception. Although a large number of corresponding points on the retinas project to corresponding cortical loci, the two of greatest concern are the foveas of the two eyes. When the visual axes (imaginary lines from the fovea through the center of the cornea) intersect at the object of regard, both foveas are stimulated by the object of regard, send impulses to corresponding areas of the cortex, and result in a single perception. If, as in the case of strabismus, the visual axes are not aligned and do not intersect at the object of regard, the object will appear doubled. Double vision (diplopia) is confusing and uncomfortable and therefore is a strong stimulus for fusion. However, if fusion does not take place, individuals will subconsciously ignore the visual input to the nonaligned eye. The eye is open, the retina is stimulated and impulses are sent to the brain, but the input is suppressed in the interest of single vision and comfort. If children with strabismus suppress vision in one eye to avoid the discomfort of diplopia, they may develop amblyopia, a condition in which the visual acuity of an eye is decreased as a result of disuse. The prognosis for improving amblyopia is dependent upon age of onset, age at which therapy is initiated, and the causative factors of the amblyopia.

In our society we are highly motivated and pressured to achieve academically. Therefore, much of what we do visually takes place at a near working distance of 13–16 inches. It is important to note the significantly higher demands of near work on the visual system. Under normal conditions, when a person looks far away the two eyes point straight ahead, the lens of the eye is at its resting state, and no adjustment is required for the two foveas to point to the same place. However, when the individual looks up close, the eyes must converge in a precise way so both foveas point to the same place to produce a single image, and the eyes must accommodate to the viewing distance so that the individual sees clearly. In reading, this relationship between accommodation and convergence must be maintained as the individual scans the lines of text. During this time, demands on accommodation and convergence are rapidly changing. Therefore accommodation and convergence must be efficient and automatic for the individual to obtain the most information while reading.

NORMAL DEVELOPMENT OF VISUAL SKILLS

Recent literature clearly supports the fact that by 6 months of age the normal infant possesses a relatively precocious visual system.

Visual Acuity

As recently as 20 years ago, it was believed that children were not physiologically capable of achieving 20/20 visual acuity until age 5–6 years. However, electrophysiological measurement of VEPs shows infants can appreciate 20/200 acuity by 6–45 days (Harter, Deaton, & Odom, 1977) and 20/20 by 6 months (Sokol & Dobson, 1976; Marg, Freeman, Peltzman, & Goldstein, 1976). Dayton et al. (1964) using OKN, found that one-day-old infants were able to respond to the 20/150 stripes. On a behavioral scale, FPL shows infants at 6 months of age able to make preference responses to stripes at an acuity value of 20/100 (Gwiazda, Brill, Mohindra, & Held, 1978; Dobson, 1980; Teller, 1981; Dobson, 1983).

Ocular Motility

Newborns show eye movements which are not random, but rather are target directed. The latencies for saccadic eye movements are longer and patterns of exploration are more erratic than the adult's; however, the target-directed saccadics are evidence of some active exploration of the visual world at birth. Fixational capture, the tendency of infants to fixate one area, occurs up to 1 month of age. As infants get older they actively begin to explore their environment. Pursuit abilities occur later than saccades. Horizontal pursuits appear first at about 2 months, vertical pursuits emerge next, and finally by 4 months the child is demonstrating circular pursuit eye movements. By 6 months of age the infant's eye movements approximate adult capability.

Accommodation

Using retinoscopy (Banks, 1980; Haynes, White, & Held, 1965) or photo-refraction (Braddick, Atkinson, French, & Howland, 1979) accommodation has been accurately measured in infants. These investigators agree that by 3 months the infant's accommodation is approaching adult capability and appropriateness. Brookman (1983) reported that accommodation decreased in accuracy during the 2nd to 8th weeks of life, and then increased in accuracy to reach adult-like proficiency at 16–20 weeks.

Vergence, Fusion, and Stereopsis

Convergence is not well established in the newborn (2–5 days old) (Wickelgren, 1967); but, by age 12–17 weeks, the infant can make vergence movements accurate enough to produce consistent fusion and a resultant

3-dimensional perception (Aslin, 1977; Fox, Aslin, Shea, & Dumais, 1980; Held, Birch, & Gwiazda, 1980; Shea, Fox, Aslin, & Dumais, 1980). The basic mechanisms which underlie biofoveal fixation and fusion are present in rudimentary form at birth. However, there are certain sensory and motor constraints that prevent them from working normally. Once these constraints are overcome, the infant demonstrates adult-like binocular functioning. This occurs between 3 and 6 months of age. Since the motor constraints which limit fusion are normal up to 5–6 months of age, it is not unusual to see a strabismus present, at times, up to this age. However, if a strabismus persists beyond this age, it should be considered abnormal, and the infant should be evaluated by an optometrist or ophthalmologist. (An *optometrist* is trained and licensed to evaluate visual function; diagnose and treat abnormalities of refraction, visual skills and visual perceptual dysfunction; diagnose ocular pathologies; and fit contact lenses. An *ophthalmologist* is a medical doctor specializing in the diagnosis and treatment of ocular pathology, as well as nonpathologic anomalies of vision.)

ANOMALIES OF VISUAL SKILLS

Ocular Motor Dysfunction

By 6 months of age, the infant has developed the ocular motor skills of pursuit and saccadic movements to near-adult levels. At this age these capabilities represent more motor than sensory performance. As a child grows, eye movements become more directly related to visual activity. For example, the younger child uses head and neck movements rather than eye movements to follow a moving target. As the child learns to separate muscle systems, eye movements replace the head/neck movements. However, some children lag in this process and continue to use head movement when it is no longer appropriate. These children have difficulty keeping their place in a book, will get to the end of one line and instead of saccading to the next line, saccade back to the beginning of the same line and reread lines. Children with poor eye movements usually have great difficulty keeping their place while reading, but finger pointing will greatly reduce this tendency. Some children can smoothly track so long as their head is allowed to move, but cannot use eye movements to track if their head is restrained. These children have the same problem with saccadic eye movements. The importance of fixational skills has been stressed. The child with poor fixational ability is likely to get inaccurate information from any stimulus.

Reading involves a lot of ocular motor activity and persons with poor ocular motor skills may have difficulty with this component of the reading process. Manifestations of ocular motor dysfunction include inability to fixate words, skipping and/or rereading lines, losing one's place frequently, finger pointing, and head movement while reading.

Fusional Instabilities

Strabismus is the extreme of a fusional problem. Another problem, called "phoria," is a *tendency* for the eye to deviate which the individual can counteract through sufficient convergence or divergence. For example, esophoria, the tendency for the eye to turn in, could be overcome by exercising the appropriate amount of divergence. Exophoria, the tendency for the eye to turn outward, could be "neutralized" with an appropriate amount of convergence. In general, people have much greater ability to converge their eyes than to diverge them. Therefore a person can deal with an exophoria more easily than an esophoria. Most of us have small phorias and therefore the convergence or divergence effort necessary to keep the eyes aligned on target is insignificant. However, as the phoria approaches the limits of the person's vergence abilities, the effort needed to keep the eyes aligned (i.e., overcome the phoria) adversely affects performance of the visual task. High phorias and/or poor vergence abilities may produce incomprehension during near visual tasks, intermittent blur, intermittent diplopia, headaches, and many other symptoms of ocular fatigue. The individual has to expend too much effort maintaining the singleness of vision and very often will *avoid* doing close work because of the discomfort which near vision tasks create.

Accommodative Insufficiency

As described earlier, younger people have the potential to make large changes in the focus of the eye due to softness of the crystalline lens. However, they are not necessarily able to effect such a change as the need arises or else must expend too much energy to produce clarity of vision at near. This does not mean that they do not have the physiological capability, but rather are unaware of how to control the ciliary muscle around the crystalline lens. Children with accommodative problems complain of blurred vision at near focus, headaches, diplopia, and/or ocular fatigue.

VISUAL PERCEPTUAL DEVELOPMENT

In simple terms perception may be viewed as the interpretation of sensations, but perception is an intricately complex process. Visual-perceptual-motor development involves the integration of visual experience with inputs from other sensory modalities, especially tactile and kinesthetic (Ayers, 1961; Banus, 1971).

Early psychologists believed that infants were incapable of perceiving. Goldstein (1980) quotes William James' comment that the world of the newborn is a "great blooming buzzing confusion." After reviewing the voluminous research on perceptual development, Goldstein notes that "while infants perceive a great deal more than James gave them credit for, they still have a long way to go before reaching adult standards of perception."

Another early view held that infants were like empty vessels waiting passively to be filled. Their passivity and "emptiness" were attributed to central nervous system immaturity. This view has been challenged by studies showing that normal neonates can be visually stimulated to imitate tongue protrusion, which is a motor act in response to visual stimulation (Meltzoff & Moore, 1983). Intermodal perception between touch and vision has been demonstrated in month-old infants and between hearing and vision in 18–20 week old infants (Kuhl & Meltzoff, 1982).

From these early beginnings perceptual skills develop rapidly. Among the factors influencing visual perceptual development are the quality of eye functions and the nature of experience. Significant visual dysfunction that may adversely affect perception is found in many children with cerebral palsy. The movement disorders and restricted mobility, characteristic of cerebral palsy, limit the child's experience. Movement is an important contributor to perceptual development and other aspects of learning (Ayres, 1961; Getman, 1962). Until infants learn to move their heads, they can only look at what is placed in front of them. With the development of movement, the infant begins to interact more with the environment. Through movement the child forms perceptions of spatial relationships which provide the basis for making many visual judgments. For accurate visual judgments, the subjective visual space (what is perceived visually by the individual) must match the objective visual space (what is physically present). Piaget and Inhelder (1956) viewed the organization of space and the eventual visual understanding of it as a developmental process. It starts from an egocentric point of view in which the child perceives only spatial relationships between self and objects in space, and progresses to encompass perceptions of relationships of objects in the environment to each other. This developmental process begins with an awareness of some constant against which other things may be referenced. Awareness of one's body provides the individual with an invariant structure against which to reference spatiality. Initial body awareness is gross, but gradually the individual becomes aware of being two-sided and of the differences between the two sides. Awareness of bilaterality is the basis for developing concepts of directionality, which are necessary for effective functioning in a society which emphasizes academic performance. Stability of directional concepts enables the individual to make accurate judgments about form and spatial relationships. The child who reverses letters and numbers may have poor directional concepts. In normal development, children reverse letters and numbers up to and including age 8. However, by 8 years of age concepts of directionality should be stable enough to prevent such errors. The important thing to watch, therefore, from 5–8 years of age is reversal frequency. As these concepts develop normally, reversal errors should decrease in frequency.

The issue of whether perceptual motor training is effective in producing improvement in academic performance is a controversial one and much too complicated to address in this chapter. However, it has been shown that perceptual motor training is effective in producing significant improvement in perceptual-motor abilities, even with controls for maturation effect (Farr & Leibowitz, 1976).

VISION IN THE CEREBRAL PALSIED CHILD

Factors which cause visual problems in the general population also operate to produce visual problems for the cerebral palsied. Because of their neuromuscular dysfunction, visual development may be disturbed in other ways. For example, some children cannot stabilize their head position; hence, their eyes never have a stable position from which to search their environment and learn clues for orientation. When neuromotor dysfunction affects eye muscles, ocular motor problems occur. Development of visual-motor skills is adversely influenced by the difficulty of coordinating direction of gaze and hand movement. Early visual development is disturbed by the motor defects. *Any* young child with a visual defect suffers an impedance of early learning experience. When this occurs in the cerebral palsied child, it is an added and confounding problem for the child (Holt & Reynell, 1967). Early detection and remediation of visual problems, therefore, are important for all children, but especially those with CP.

Ocular-Motor Disorders

Studies of visual problems in the cerebral palsied child point to a significantly higher incidence of visual anomalies in this population. Probably because of differences in the nature of the groups studied, there is a large variance in incidence data. In the general population of normal children, ages 6–17 years, the incidence of strabismus ranges between 5.5% and 6.7% (Altman, Hiatt, & Deweese, 1966; Roberts, 1972). In an approximately equivalent age range of cerebral palsied children, the percentages range from as low as 15% to as high as 60% (see Table 6.1).

Pigassou-Albuoy and Fleming (1975) suggest that the high incidence of strabismus, with a breakdown in binocular vision, in the CP population is the result of lesions in the motor centers of the brain. These lesions could easily affect elaboration of higher cortical processes of which binocular vision is just one. They further hypothesize that the difficulty in curing strabismus (and amblyopia) in this population occurs because a significant component of the strabismus is neurological in nature and not "uniquely functional" as in normal children. The frequent occurrence of strabismus in CP has focused attention on this particular visual finding, often to the exclusion of others. However, some studies of CP children have found high percentages of other problems, such as significant refractive error and amblyopia. Duckman (1979) found ocular motor dysfunction in 92% of a group of 25 cerebral palsied children, and all of them had accommodative insufficiency. These data are all significantly higher than those published by the U.S. Department of Health, Education and Welfare through the Vital and Health Statistic Surveys of normal children (Roberts, 1978).

TABLE 6.1
Prevalence of Visual Anomalies in Cerebral Palsied Children

Researcher(s)	N	ST*	AB*	O-M*	V-P*	AC*	E*
Guibor (1953)	147	60	25				
Breakey (1955)	100	48					
Schrire (1956)	73	15					
Lossef (1962)	88	34					67
Wiesinger (1964)	75	51					40
Altman et al. (1966)	64	44	6				76
Jones & Dayton (1968)	28	60					
Breakey et al. (1968	120	44	23				
Pearlstone & Benjamin (1969)	30	40					
Levy et al. (1976)	108	17					
Duckman (1979)	25	56		92	78	100	40
Black (1980)	117	51	15				
Scheiman (1984)	73	69					64

*ST — Strabismus
 AB — Amblyopia
 O-M — Ocular motor dysfunction
 V-P — Visual perceptual dysfunction
 AC — Accommodation
 E   — Significant refractive error

N — The N value for each of the above studies was either the number of consecutive cerebral palsied children examined or, in retrospective studies, the number of patient records examined.

Spastics are more likely to have visual defects than athetoids. Hiles, Waller, and McFarlane (1975) found that of a group of cerebral palsied persons with strabismus, 85% were spastic and only 15% athetoid. Breakey, Wilson, and Wilson (1968) found that both spastics and athetoids differed significantly from a nonneurologically involved control group. Table 6.2 summarizes some of their data.

TABLE 6.2
Incidence of Visual Defects (In Percentage)

DEFECT	SPASTIC (N = 60)	ATHETOID (N = 60)	CONTROL (N = 60)
Refractive Error	64	35	32
Acuity of 20/40 or Less	24	12	0
Optic Atrophy	7	2	0
Amblyopia	28	16	2
Strabismus	60	28	8

Perceptual Disorders

It has long been recognized that perceptual difficulties may be a direct result of brain damage in children (Strauss & Lehtinen, 1947; Cruickshank, Bice, Wallen, & Lynch, 1957). In addition there is the possibility of a relationship between visual dysfunction and perceptual deficits. Abercrombie (1960) stated that if eye movements are "uncoordinated, jerky or slow, the fixation periods too long or too short, the sequence of images received on the retina will be abnormal and difficulties of integrating them into meaningful perceptions may be increased." Another possible cause of perceptual disorders in cerebral palsy is the disruption of movement which is characteristic of the condition. Earlier in this chapter we noted that restricted motility limits the child's opportunities to gain experiences which are essential for perceptual development. There is also the possibility that movement is directly related to perceptual development.

The relationship between motor handicaps and perceptual-motor performance in CP has not been well established. However, Piaget (1956), Kephart (1960), Getman (1962), and Gesell, Ilg, and Bullis (1979), among others, emphasize the importance of movement in establishing visuospatial concepts. This does not suggest that CP children, with restricted motor ability, will not develop these concepts, but rather that the lack of motor experience necessitates the use of alternate strategies in such conceptual development. These alternate strategies, however, require higher intellectual functioning to recognize the need and then develop the strategy. It appears that if restricted movement patterns do not prevent development of perceptual concepts, they do retard the process. This could account for the high frequency of visual perception dysfunction in children with severe motor handicaps. Wedell, Newman, Reid, and Bradbury (1972) reported that limited experience of independent mobility is significantly associated with reduction in size constancy in CP children. Size constancy is a spatial perceptual constancy which allows the individual to understand that an object maintains a constant physical size despite variations of retinal image size as the object moves to different distances from the observer. Wedell's experiment does not provide conclusive proof that lack of motor experience deters perceptual and cognitive development, but it suggests, along with the high incidence of perceptual-motor dysfunction in this population, that lack of motor experience may be a causative factor in delayed perceptual development.

There are indications that disturbances of figure-ground perception and visual perceptual-motor functions are more common in cerebral palsy than in nonhandicapped children; however, there is large variation among subjects of similar chronological age. Generally spastics are more likely than athetoids to exhibit problems in these areas (Cruickshank, Bice, Wallen, & Lynch, 1965).

REMEDIATION AND THERAPY

While much has been written about visual problems in CP, there has been little published about remediation of these problems. In three papers (Duckman, 1980, 1984, 1985) I have discussed some aspects of remediation in a population of severely involved CP children. It is my feeling that if change in visual function can be effected in this population, it should be more easily effected in a less severely involved group of CPs.

In the treatment of visual problems of cerebral palsied children, it is important to define carefully the full scope of visual deficits, and evaluate how the visual problems might affect performance. After determining which deficits can be remediated, goals and objectives should be outlined, and an appropriate treatment plan designed. Visual therapy must be integrated with other therapies to produce the best results and to aid in fulfilling the objectives of other therapy programs.

The goal of any therapy program should be to effect change in a positive direction. To do this, the therapist must begin at an appropriate level of difficulty. If the task is too simple, the child will usually perform with little to no conscious effort. If it is too difficult, the child will give up. In either case, change will not occur. Therefore it is important to start at a level where the child is challenged, but with conscious effort can be successful.

It is important to keep in mind that progress with these children is *slow*. Therefore, it is advisable for the therapist and for the child that goals be well-defined, *realistic* and *short-term*. Whenever possible, positive rein-forcement schedules should be employed to strengthen the child's moti-vation for working at the task. In the section below, various visual activities are described. In selecting tasks for training, the therapist must consider the child's visual limitations. For example, a child who cannot see a target should not be expected to follow that target during an ocular motility activity. Working on saccadic eye movements would be inappropriate for the child who cannot move the eye to either side, or up or down because of an EOM paresis or paralysis. Regardless of how long and hard the child tries, the task cannot be performed successfully. A child with an accom-modative problem should not be given tasks which demand accommoda-tive ability. A child with optic atrophy, who cannot achieve visual acuity, may be *best* served by using magnifiers, and/or large presentations rather than through ocular or perceptual motor activities.

Ocular Motor Activities

Ocular motor activities are indicated when children have poor fixational skills, and/or poor pursuit and saccadic ability because these skills are essential for many educational activities and for using communication aids. Education and communication goals may be easier to achieve once the goals of visual therapy are met.

General Considerations.   To optimize the child's chance of succeed-ing, many factors should receive attention before visual training is begun.

Positioning.   A child who cannot follow a moving target sitting up, may be able to do so if laid in a supine position. Sitting, the child must exert different amounts of effort as the eyes move down and up (toward and against the pull of gravity), but in a supine position, with head straight up toward the ceiling, the effort is the same in all directions.

Environment.   A child will have an easier time following and fixat-ing a target if there is a minimum of interfering stimuli. A large illumi-nated room with many stimuli (referred to as noise) is more distracting than a small, darkened, empty one.

Head Movements.   Ultimately the child should be able to follow a target using eye movements only, but initially allowing the child to use head movements to follow moving targets will set up the foundations for a fovea-to-target match. Then as the skills improve, an attempt should be made to minimize head movement by using sandbags if the child is supine and holding the head if the child is sitting.

Presenting Targets. Practice is required to learn at what speed targets should be moved. The eye can track at a maximum velocity of about 20 degrees/second, but children with poor pursuit skills will track much more slowly. It is better to move the target too slowly than too quickly. To maintain interest, activities should be changed frequently and "boring" activities should be intermingled with "fun" ones. Even with a child whose attention span is short, attempts at tracking are worth the effort.

Monocular and Binocular Tracking. Initially, training should be given to one eye at a time. This is done by using an eye patch during the activity. It is critical that the eye patch be used only during monocular training and removed immediately thereafter. The therapist should work toward equality of monocular performance (i.e., right eye performance should approximately equal left eye performance). Therefore, if one eye seems to be doing better at a particular task, greater time should be spent practicing with the poorer eye. When the two eyes have equal and adequate performance skills, an attempt can be made to do the activity binocularly (assuming binocularity exists) or increase the difficulty of the monocular task.

Training Activities. The following are ordered in degree of difficulty from least difficult:

Tube Rotations. When no other task can be achieved, put the child supinely on a mat, in a totally darkened room. Hold one end of a cylinder, such as an empty paper towel tube, to one eye. At the other end of the tube present a flashlight. Keeping one end close to the eye, slowly rotate the other end in a circular motion. If the tube is held close to the eye and the only stimulus available to the child is the light, then as the tube is moved the child will follow the target. Often the use of colored filters or translucent finger puppets over the flashlight will hold the child's interest longer. As the eye starts to follow better, slowly move the tube away from the eye, eventually removing the tube entirely. Then present the flashlight without out the tube in a darkened room and gradually increase room illumination so the child ultimately can follow the target in a normally illuminated room with peripheral "noise" present. As the tube is eliminated, the movement of the target can take on random patterns or specific patterns such as circumscribing letters of the alphabet for the child to identify. As the skill improves, the target can be changed from a flashlight to a finger puppet, to a racing car moving on a track, to a computer generated object, or to any target which will enhance fixation and pursuit eye movement. Tactile stimulation (have the child touch the target as it is being moved) often helps increase the accuracy of the eye movements and the duration of fixation.

Mirror Rotations. This can be done in either a sitting or supine position. The target for fixation and pursuit is the child's own eye. A small mirror is held in front of one eye (about 13–16 inches away) and the child is instructed to watch the eye as the therapist slowly moves the mirror while watching the child's eye. Verbal feedback should be given whenever the child's eye is not fixating appropriately.

Swinging Yarn Ball. From a distance of about 3 to 4 feet, and at eye level, have the child monocularly follow a target, such as a yarn ball suspended from a string as it moves in a pendular motion. A variation of this activity for those children with adequate hand control, is to swing the yarn ball toward and away from them and let them try to hit the ball in such a way that it hits the therapist (i.e., the child must "aim for" the therapist).

The Spelling Flashlight. The therapist and the child face a blank wall in a darkened room. The therapist holds a flashlight and slowly moves it as if writing capital letters. After each letter, the child is asked to describe what was "printed" on the wall. Depending on the child's ability, the therapist can "print" single letters or numbers, simple shapes, simple vocabulary words or simple sentences (one letter at a time).

Racetrack Motility. This can be done as a pursuit movement activity or combined to integrate hand-eye coordination, depending on the child's motor ability. Draw a racetrack on the blackboard as illustrated in Figure 6.2. Begin with a simple oval with the center filled in and progress to more complex tracks. Either the therapist or the child may hold a flashlight. If the therapist holds the flashlight, the child's task is to pretend that the light is a car and visually follow it as it rides around the road. If the light goes off the road (and the therapist should allow this to happen), the child must indicate that this has happened. A child who can manipulate the flashlight does the driving and tries to keep the car on the road.

Follow the Leader. This can be done only with children who are able to manipulate a flashlight. With the child and therapist each holding a flashlight, the therapist slowly moves one light around on a blank wall and the child tries to keep his or her light on top of the therapist's light so that at all times only one light is seen. It is helpful to put colored filters in front of the flashlights so that the child's light can be differentiated from the therapist's.

Groffman Tracking. On a blackboard in front of the child at eye level, the therapist draws a set of symbols placed vertically on the left side of the board and an equivalent number of different symbols on the right side of the board. Then "squiggly" lines are drawn from the symbols on the left side to the symbols on the right side as illustrated in Figure 6.3. The degree of difficulty is dependent on the number of symbols used, the complexity of the path going from left to right, and the number of intersections created. The symbols may be numbers, letters, geometric shapes, or pictures of familiar objects. The child's task is to follow the path from one symbol on the left and tell the therapist to which symbol on the right it leads.

Record Player Pursuits. For this activity a children's record player with variable speeds (use the slowest speed to start) and removable cover is needed. Make cardboard "records" about the size of a long playing disk. Begin with only one colored circle about the size of a quarter on the record. The following tracking activities utilize these materials: the child follows the colored circle while the therapist watches the eye movements; the child

SIMPLE

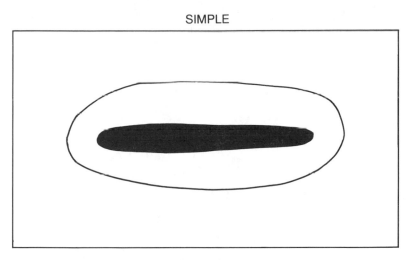

COMPLEX

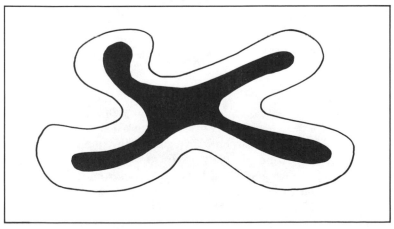

Figure 6.2. Racetrack motility.

keeps a small flashlight directed on the circle as it spins around; the therapist holds the flashlight on the circle and the child indicates whenever the light is not on the circle; the child holds a pencil or crayon and on the command of the therapist moves the pencil or crayon to "hit" the circle. As this skill improves, the therapist can add more circles. If the child has the skills, the therapist can put many circles on the record, and put letters and/or numbers in the circles. The child spells words by bringing the pencil into the appropriate circle, one letter at a time, while the disk is rotating. If numbers are placed in the circles, the therapist can have the child do math problems such as selecting two numbers which add up to 12. In this way educational goals can be achieved at the same time that ocular motilities are being improved. Of course, the latter activity can only be practiced if the child has the intellectual capacity to perform the task.

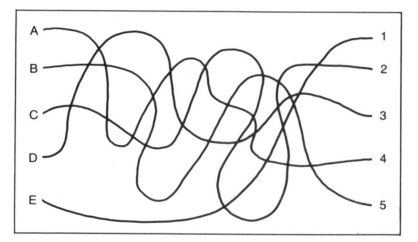

Figure 6.3. Groffman track.

Training Saccadic Movements.   Saccadic eye movements are important for the child who uses communication aids for reading and classroom activities. The following activities will improve saccadic movements:

Finding Objects.   With the child in a sitting position, stabilize the head and say to the child "find with your eye(s)" as you name different objects in the room. The therapist should watch the movement of the eye(s) as it searches for the named object. An especially effective way to do this is to place the child about 2 feet from a large mirror. By standing behind the child, the therapist can now observe the child's eyes and the objects in the room behind them.

Blackboard Saccadics.   Seat the child facing a blackboard at eye level at a distance of about 3 to 4 feet. In each corner of the blackboard place a figure or a picture of a familiar object. The therapist kneels, facing the child, between the blackboard and the child, but below the child's line of sight. Instruct the child to look at the appropriate picture as the therapist names, in random order, those pictures placed on the board. If the child has no difficulty locating four pictures located in the corners, increase the number by placing additional pictures around the periphery of the board. It is helpful if you have a small diagram of what you've placed on the board so you don't have to keep turning around to find out if the child is correct. To increase the difficulty of the task, code each picture on the periphery of the blackboard with a number and write several numbers in the center of the board as in Figure 6.4. The child reads a number in the center of the board and then looks at the appropriately numbered item on the board. The therapist must stand in front of the child and observe the eye movements to ensure that the task is being done correctly.

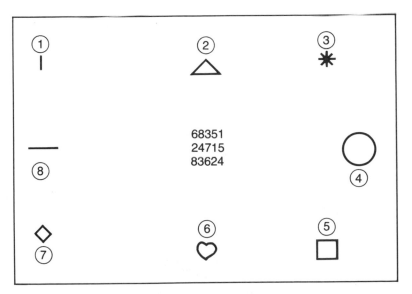

Figure 6.4. Blackboard saccadics with coding.

Grid Activities.   Arrange pictures of familiar objects, words, or symbols in a 2 x 2 matrix. Code each row with a color or letter and each column with a number or shape as in Figure 6.5. When the therapist names one of the symbols, the child finds it and uses the code to indicate the row and column intersection. The therapist might vary this task by naming a row and a column and having the child identify which symbol is in the box. The number of cells in the matrix may be increased gradually as the child improves.

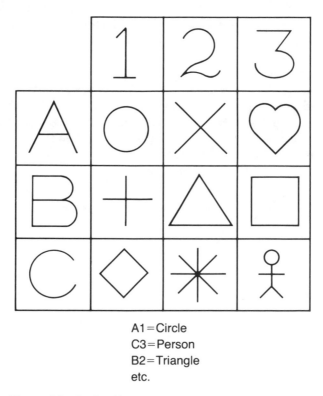

A1 = Circle
C3 = Person
B2 = Triangle
etc.

Figure 6.5. 3 x 3 grid.

Cops and Robbers. This activity can be used only with a child who has enough hand control to manipulate a flashlight. It should be done monocularly in either a totally or partially darkened room. The therapist, playing robber, and the child, playing cop, each hold a flashlight and face a blank wall. The task is for the child (cop) to catch the therapist (robber) who has just taken one of the child's favorite possessions. As in the "Follow the Leader" activity, the therapist's light is flashed on the wall and the child tries to put his or her light directly on it, so that the two lights superimpose. The therapist immediately and rapidly moves the light to another spot on the wall, and the child must keep catching it. As soon as the two lights are superimposed, the therapist once again rapidly moves the light.

Accommodation and Vergence Training

While accommodation activities are important to this population, these are best accomplished by the use of lenses. Therefore it is necessary to have supervision of these activities by an appropriate health professional. This is also true of activities which increase vergence and fusional skills.

Perceptual-Motor Activities

Several disciplines, particularly special education, occupational therapy, psychology, and optometry, have been interested in perceptual-motor functions. The following are examples of activities designed to improve perceptual-motor function.

Body Awareness. Being aware of one's body is essential to the understanding of directional concepts. Body part identification games with lots of movement and touch to reinforce and provide feedback are helpful. If the child has sufficient control of body parts, "Touch and Go" is a good activity. With the child supine on the floor, the therapist touches a part of the body and asks the child to move "only the part(s) touched" a predetermined amount. For example: "If I touch your arm I want you to move it to shoulder level. If I touch your leg I want you to move it out 2 feet." In order of difficulty, try (from the simplest): both arms *or* both legs; one arm *or* one leg; arm *and* leg of same side; arm *and* leg of opposite sides. Most CP children do not have enough independent movement to do these tasks, so the therapist may move the body parts for the child in an attempt to build awareness.

Directional Concepts.

Rote Memory of Right/Left. The use of markers on hands or shoes can help the child learn the labels *right* and *left*. However, these markers should be referenced against something on the child's body, rather than against external objects so that the child begins to understand the referencing of direction. For example, if you tell the child that his/her right arm is on the same side as the window, then when the child is in another room or in another position he/she may continue to reference "right" to the position of the window. Identification games are also helpful: "Show me your right hand; show me your left eye; show me your left ear; show me your right knee." This activity also builds body awareness.

Directional Arrows. Make a series of arrows on the blackboard. (Perhaps 4 rows of 4 each with the 16 arrows facing random directions.) The child starts at the top left and "reads" the arrows in order, naming the directions of each. At first, the arrows should face up, down, left, or right, but later on the four oblique directions can be added (i.e., up and right, up and left, down and right, down and left).

Directional Maps. Make simple line maps using vertical and horizontal lines at first. The map should show a starting position and lead to some place the child would like to go. Then the child verbally gives the therapist instructions on how to move a pencil to travel the road which has been drawn. The child must watch as the therapist traces over the lines and tell the therapist to stop at all turns, and which way to go from each "corner." If the child gives incorrect directions, the therapist should follow the child's command by going the wrong way and continuing until the child says "Stop!" Now the child must give directions to return to the point where the error was made and proceed from there. If the child doesn't say "Stop!" at a corner, the therapist should continue until the child realizes the error; then the child must direct the therapist back to the corner. In this way the child learns to track carefully and give verbal instructions about directionality at the same time. As the child begins to improve, slowly, oblique lines can be introduced to the map.

Moving Around in Space. The therapist and the child actually move around the environment on the basis of the child's verbal instructions. This can be done while the child is in a wheelchair or with a walker.

Form Perception (Size and Shape). At the lowest level, form board puzzles may be utilized. Incorporate verbal output so that the child must describe the activity. Have the child name the shape and/or tell in which hole the piece belongs. Encourage the use of vision to identify the correct placement rather than trial and error placement. Encourage tactile reinforcement of the pieces and the holes. As the child becomes more adept at placing pieces in form boards, use simple parquetry block designs. This is an effective technique when combined with verbal instructions. Start out with two squares and work up to combinations of square and triangle, square and diamond, triangle and diamond, etc. Encourage the child to describe what is being done as it is being done. For example, if you show the child a red square to the left side of a green square, the child must explain either that there is a red square to the left of a green square, or the green square is to the right of the red square. If the child does not know right from left, saying the green is to the side of the red or vice versa is sufficient. Increase the degree of difficulty by increasing the number of pieces you are working with at any given time.

For additional ideas and activities see Smith and Cote (1982) and Getman (1962). An optometric program in a school for cerebral palsied children is described in Duckman (1985).

REFERENCES

Abercrombie, M. L. J. (1960). Perception and eye movements: Some speculations on disorders in cerebral palsy. *Cerebral Palsy Bulletin, 2*, 142–148.

Altman, H. E., Hiatt, R. L., & Deweese, M. W. (1966). Ocular findings in cerebral palsy. *Southern Medical Journal, 59*, 1015–1018.

Aslin, R. (1977). Development of binocular fixation in human infants. *Journal of Exceptional Child Psychology, 23*, 133–150.

Ayers, A. J. (1961). The role of gross-motor activities in the training of children with visual-motor retardation. *Journal of the American Optometric Association, 33*(2), 121–125.

Banks, M. S. (1980). The development of visual accommodation during early infancy. *Child Development, 51*, 546–566.

Banus, B. S. (1971). *The developmental therapist.* Thorofare, NJ: Charles B. Slack.

Black, P. D. (1980). Ocular defects in children with cerebral palsy. *British Medical Journal, 281*, 484–488.

Braddick, O. J., Atkinson, J., French, J., & Howland, H. C. (1979). A photorefractive study of infant accommodation. *Vision Research, 19*, 1319–1330.

Breakey, A. S. (1955). Ocular findings in cerebral palsy. *Archives Ophthalmology, 53*, 852–856.

Breakey, A. S., Wilson, J., & Wilson, B. C. (1968). The relationship between visual disorders and visual perception deficits in cerebral palsy. *Developmental Medicine and Child Neurology, 10*(2), 251–252.

Brookman, K. E. (1983). Ocular accommodation in human infants. *American Journal of Optometry and Physiologic Optics, 60*(2), 91–99.

Cruickshank, W. M., Bice, H. V., Wallen, N. E., & Lynch, K. (1957). *Perception and cerebral palsy.* Syracuse, NY: Syracuse University Press.

Cruickshank, W. M., Bice, H. V., Wallen, N. E., & Lynch, K. (1965). *Perception and cerebral palsy* (2nd ed.). Syracuse, NY: Syracuse University Press.

Davidson, S. I. (1974). *Aspects of neuro-ophthalmology.* London: Butterworth and Company.

Dayton, G. O., Jr., Jones, M. H., Aiu, P., Rawson, R. A., Steele, B., & Rose, M. (1964). Developmental study of coordinated eye movements in the human infant—I. Visual acuity in the newborn human. *Archives Ophthalmology, 48*, 721–730.

Dobson, V. (1980). Behavioral tests of visual acuity in infants. *International Ophthalmology Clinic, 20*(1), 233–250.

Dobson, V. (1983). Clinical applications of preferential looking measures of visual acuity. *Behavior Brain Research, 10*, 25–38.

Duckman, R. H. (1979). Incidence of visual anomalies in a population of cerebral palsied children. *Journal of the American Optometric Association, 50*(9), 1013–1016.

Duckman, R. H. (1980). Effectiveness of visual training on a population of cerebral palsied children. *Journal of the American Optometric Association, 51*(6), 607–614.

Duckman, R. H. (1984). Accommodation in cerebral palsy: Function and remediation. *Journal of the American Optometric Association, 55*(4), 281–283.

Duckman, R. H. (1984). Effectiveness of optometric visual training in a population of severely involved cerebral palsied children utilizing professional, non-optometric therapists. *Physical and Occupational Therapy in Pediatrics, 4*(4), 75–86.

Duckman, R. H., & Selenow, A. (1983). Visual acuity in neurologically impaired children. *American Journal of Optometry and Physiologic Optics, 60*(10), 817–21.

Fantz, R. L. (1958). Pattern vision in young infants. *Psychological Record, 8*, 43–47.

Farr, J., & Leibowitz, H. W. (1976). An experimental study of the efficacy of perceptual-motor training. *American Journal of Optometry and Physiologic Optics, 53*(9), 451–455.

Fox, R., Aslin, R. N., Shea, S. L., & Dumais, S. T. (1980). Stereopsis in human infants. *Science, 207,* 232–324.

Gesell, A., Ilg, F. L., & Bullis, G. E. (1979). *Vision—Its development in infant and child.* New York: Paul Hoeber, Inc.

Getman, G. N. (1962). *How to improve your child's intelligence.* Published privately, Luverne, MN.

Goldstein, E. B. (1980). *Sensation and perception.* Belmont, CA: Wadsworth.

Guibor, G. P. (1953). Some eye defects seen in cerebral palsy. *American Journal of Physical Medicine, 32,* 342–347.

Gwiazda, J., Brill, S., Mohindra, I., & Held, R. (1978). Infant visual acuity and its meridional variation. *Vision Research, 18,* 1469–1483.

Harter, M. R., Deaton, F. K., & Odom, J. V. (1977). Maturation of evoked potentials and visual preference in 6–45-day old infants: Effects of check size, visual acuity and refractive error. *Electroencephalography Clinical Neurophysiology, 42*(5), 595–607.

Haynes, H., White, B. L., & Held, R. (1965). Visual accommodation in human infants. *Science, 148,* 528–530.

Held, R., Birch, E., & Gwiazda, J. (1980). Stereoacuity of human infants. *Proceedings of the National Academy of Science, USA, 77,* 5572–5574.

Hiles, D. A., Waller, P. H., & McFarlane, F. (1975). Current concepts in the management of strabismus in children with cerebral palsy. *Annals Ophthalmology, 7*(6), 789–798.

Holt, K. S., & Reynell, J. K. (1967). *Assessment of cerebral palsy—Volume II.* London: Lloyd-Duke.

Jones, M. H., & Dayton, G. O. (1968). Assessment of visual disorders in cerebral palsy. *Archives of Italian Pediatrics, 25*(3), 251–264.

Kephart, N. (1960). *The slow learner in the classroom.* Chicago: Merrill.

Kuhl, P. K., & Meltzoff, A. N. (1982). The bimodal perception of speech in infancy. *Science, 218,* 1138–1141.

Levy, N. S., Cassin, B., & Newman, M. (1976). Strabismus in children with cerebral palsy. *Journal of Pediatric Ophthalmology, 13*(2), 72–74.

Lossef, S. (1962). Ocular findings in cerebral palsy. *American Journal of Ophthalmology, 54*(6), 1114–1118.

Marg, E., Freeman, D. N., Peltzman, P., & Goldstein, P. J. (1976). Visual acuity development in human infants: Evoked potential measurements. *Investigative Ophthalmology, 14*(2), 150–153.

Meltzoff, A. N., & Moore, M. K. (1983). Newborn infants imitate adult facial gestures. *Child Development, 54,* 702–709.

Mueller, C., & Rudolph, M. (1970). *Light and vision.* New York: Life Science Library, Time Life Books.

Pearlstone, A., & Benjamin, R. (1969). Ocular defects in cerebral palsy. *Eye, Ear, Nose and Throat Monthly, 48*(7), 437–439.

Piaget, J., & Inhelder, B. (1956). *The child's conception of space.* London: Routledge and Kegan Paul.

Pigassou-Albuoy, R., & Fleming, A. (1975). Amblyopia and strabismus in patients with cerebral palsy. *Annals of Ophthalmology, 7*(3), 382–384 and 386–387.

Roberts, J. (1972). Eye examination findings among children. *Vital and Health Statistics, U.S. Department of HEW, 11*(115), 3–6.

Roberts, J. (1978). Refraction status and motility defects of persons 4–74 years. *Vital and Health Statistics, U.S. Department of HEW, 11*(206), 6–7; 34–36.

Schapero, M., Cline, D., & Hofstetter, H. W. (1968). *Dictionary of visual science*. Radnor, PA: Chilton Book Company.

Scheiman, M. (1984). Optometric findings in children with cerebral palsy. *American Journal of Optometry and Physiologic Optics, 61*(5), 321–323.

Schrire, L. (1956). An ophthalmological survey of a series of cerebral palsy cases. *South African Medical Journal, 30*(17), 405–407.

Shea, S. L., Fox, R., Aslin, R. N., & Dumais, S. T. (1980). Assessment of stereopsis in human infants. *Investigative Ophthalmology Vision Science, 19*, 1400–1404.

Smith, A. J., & Cote, K. S. (1982). *Look at me: A resource manual for the development of residual vision in multiply impaired children*. Philadelphia, PA: Pennsylvania College of Optometry Press.

Sokol, S., & Dobson, V. (1976). Pattern reversal visually evoked potentials in infants. *Investigative Ophthalmology, 15*(1), 58–62.

Strauss, A. A., & Lehtinen, L. (1947). *Psychopathology and education in the brain injured child*. New York: Grune and Stratton.

Teller, D. Y. (1979). The forced-choice preferential looking procedure: A psychophysical technique for use with human infants. *Infant Behavior Development, 2*, 135–153.

Teller, D. Y. (1981). The development of visual acuity in human and monkey infants. *Trends Neuroscience, 4*, 21–24.

Wedell, K., Newman, C. V., Reid, P., & Bradbury, I. R. (1972). An exploratory study of the relationship between size constancy and experience of mobility in cerebral palsied children. *Developmental Medicine and Child Neurology, 14*, 615–620.

Wertenbaker, L. (1981). *The eye: Window to the world*. Washington, D.C.: U.S. News Books.

Wickelgren, L. (1967). Convergence in the human newborn. *Journal of Exceptional Child Psychology, 5*, 74–85.

Wiesinger, H. (1964). Ocular findings in mentally retarded children. *Journal Pediatric Ophthalmology, 1*(3), 37–41.

CHAPTER 7

Prespeech and Feeding Development

Rona Alexander

Alexander takes the position that respiratory, phonatory, and oral-motor development are related to factors such as general movement development and muscular activity developed in response to weightshift. Many of the abnormal patterns which interfere with feeding and speech production she sees as movements or postures developed to compensate for abnormal postural tone, an abnormal quality of extension, and poor control of antigravity flexion. Effective treatment strategies must reflect the relationship between general antigravity movement development and the development of functional prespeech movement components.

1. *Discuss the significance of the progression from physiological flexion to active coordinated antigravity extension and flexion for development of each of the following: (a) suckling movements, (b) coordinated sucking, (c) active removal of food from a spoon, (d) abdominal/thoracic breathing, and (e) production of sounds.*
2. *Why do many children with cerebral palsy develop a pattern of head/neck hyperextension, tongue retraction, and humeral extension/adduction, and how does this abnormal pattern affect (a) respiration, (b) feeding, and (c) sound production?*
3. *How would you reconcile the view that speech production is controlled by neurophysiologic mechanisms which are distinct from the mechanisms involved in vegetative acts, and Alexander's emphasis on developing oral-motor functioning for feeding as prerequisites to later speech training?*

SIGNIFICANT ASPECTS OF PRESPEECH
AND FEEDING DEVELOPMENT

Basic to the use of efficient, intelligible speech for communication is the development of well-organized systems of oral and respiratory-phonatory motor control which is directly influenced by a variety of factors including general movement development. Every movement produced by an individual requires that there be a point of stability as well as a point of mobility in the body. This balance of active mobility and stability develops as we learn to use our musculature actively to respond to shifts of weight through anterior, posterior, lateral, and diagonal planes of movement. Although generally discussed in terms of the development of righting and equilibrium reactions, musculature activity developed in response to weightshift includes that which directly affects, and is directly affected by, oral-motor and respiratory-phonatory development.

Normal Oral-Motor Development in Feeding

The Newborn.   Passive or physiological flexion maintains the limbs of the full-term newborn flexed and adducted to the body and the head positioned with the chin against the upper chest in supine and prone (Peiper, 1963). When tactile stimulation is presented to parts of the oral area, the newborn may respond with a *rooting response*[1] *gag response*, or *automatic phasic bite-release pattern.*

During the first 2 weeks of life, the newborn takes in liquids using a total pattern of sucking activity. However, unlike the true negative-pressure *sucking* seen later in development, this total pattern of sucking activity appears directly related to the physiological flexion which biomechanically restricts jaw movement, the extremely small intraoral space which limits tongue mobility, and the positional stability of the cheeks provided by the sucking pads which maintains the lips in a more forward position around the nipple (Bosma, 1972, 1978).

As the infant begins to use head and neck extension against gravity, the chin moves away from the chest and the mandible depresses, bringing the tongue forward and downward. This new head, neck, jaw, and tongue activity results in the introduction of active *suckling* movements. Although suckling is the infant's predominant active oral pattern, sucking movements still occur when the head is held in a more stable, flexed position during bottledrinking and breastfeeding.

Rhythmical forward-backward movements of the tongue and easy tongue protrusion are used in swallowing. As the liquid travels posteriorly over the cupped tongue, movements of the back of the tongue, soft

---

[1]Terms in italics are defined at the end of the chapter.

palate, and posterior pharyngeal wall propel it back around the high-positioned epiglottis and down into the esophagus. The newborn can breathe and swallow at the same time without choking.

One to Six Months. General movement development is extensive during this period as physiological flexion decreases, active antigravity extension increases, and active antigravity flexion develops to balance with the antigravity extension. By the end of the 6th month, the infant is responding to weightshift with more active antigravity movements which help to establish a musculature base for greater fine-motor oral activities. However, it is important to note that the development of greater fine-motor oral activities results in the more active use of musculature which is not only required for progress in oral-pharyngeal-laryngeal functioning, but also plays a significant role in the infant's development of active antigravity head flexion; neck elongation; and active mobility and stability at the shoulder girdle, pelvis, and hips.

Through 4 months of age there is significant integration of the oral-tactile sensory system noted in the reduction of the rooting response and the automatic phasic bite-release pattern. Although suckling continues to be the predominant active oral-motor pattern, sucking activity increases as the infant begins to use the center portion of the lips to hold the nipple. Longer sequences of sucking or suckling are produced before the infant pauses to swallow and breathe.

Infants may be introduced to spoonfeeding, solid foods, and cupdrinking at 5 and 6 months of age. Suckling is the active pattern used initially in all of these activities. The 6-month-old child may begin to raise and protrude the lower lip under the spoon or cup, using it as a point of stability. This results in the depression of the upper lip and its posturing to assist in food removal and liquid intake. However, as the feeding utensil is removed and the lower lip no longer has a surface on which to stabilize, suckling is used to move the food or liquid back for swallowing.

As solids are presented to the infant at the front of the mouth, active suckling, sucking, or rhythmical up and down jaw movements may be used. However, solids placed on the side gums are often handled using a *munching* pattern. Coughing, choking, and gagging often occur since solid food textures provide new tactile experiences for the infant. As the infant learns to tolerate these new solid textures, choking decreases and the strength of the gag response reduces.

Seven to Twelve Months. By 8 months of age, the child has developed all of the essential movement components from which more refined, coordinated activity can be developed including increased control of weightshifting, greater dissociation of arm and leg movements, greater abdominal musculature activity, increased active trunk elongation, and greater spinal rotation within the trunk. The further integration of these movement components is reflected in the increased coordination of the 12-month-old whose new and more complex movements provide a more integrated base of neuromotor and sensory-motor activity on which greater oral-motor coordination can be established.

Coordinated sucking movements are now predominant during bottle-drinking and breastfeeding. As cheek and lip activity increase and suck-ing, swallowing, and breathing are better coordinated, liquid loss is reduced. By 9 months of age musculature activity at the cheeks and lip corners has increased so that active, complete closure around the nipple is used, and liquid loss is no longer noted.

Although coordinated sucking activity is predominant in bottle-drinking and breastfeeding by 9 months of age, suckling continues to be the primary oral pattern used in cupdrinking. It is not until approximately 10 months that the child begins to use more sucking movements actively in the cupdrinking process. Coordination of suckling or sucking, swallow-ing, and breathing is controlled as the child stops drinking or pulls away from the cup after taking two or three sucks.

In order to compensate for excessive jaw activity, the 10- to 11-month-old may begin to protrude the tongue under the cup, wrapping the lower lip around it for stability. By 13 to 15 months of age, external *jaw stabili-zation* is often achieved by biting on the cup rim so that the lips and tongue can be more actively involved in the cupdrinking process. This system of external jaw stabilization may be used until about 24 months, when greater internal jaw musculature activity has been developed.

The active removal of food from a spoon begins at approximately 7 months as the child elevates and protrudes the lower lip and lowers and protrudes the upper lip as the spoon is placed in the mouth. By 12 months the child removes food from a spoon using a highly coordinated sequence of movement components including active head flexion, neck elongation, shoulder girdle depression, trunk elongation, forward and backward hip mobility, graded depression and elevation of the jaw, active tongue stabil-ity, downward and forward/backward upper lip activity, and upward and forward/backward lower lip activity. Sucking is used to move the semi-solid food back in the mouth for swallowing.

Jaw activity in biting continues to be composed of small vertical phasic bite-release movements until approximately 8 months of age. At that time the child begins to close the jaw and posture on a cracker or soft solid, allow-ing for a piece to be broken off for chewing. A more *controlled, sustained bite* through a soft solid may be used by approximately 10 months, although it may not be used on a hard solid until 12 to 13 months of age.

Tongue movements are the first to modify at 7 months of age as *chew-ing* develops. When food is placed on the biting surfaces of the side gums, horizontal shifts or gross rolling movements of the tongue are produced.

Since there is no tongue-jaw dissociation, the jaw moves laterally and slightly diagonally as the tongue shifts horizontally. Food in the center of the mouth is handled using sucking or suckling activity.

By 10 months, with tongue movements used more actively to transfer food from the side-to-center and the center-to-side of the mouth, jaw movements change to include up/down, forward/back, and circular-lateral/ diagonal excursions. As *tongue lateralization* with side-to-side movements becomes more coordinated at 12 to 15 months, greater circular-diagonal movements of the jaw are noted. The well coordinated use of *rotary jaw movement* with refined grinding and shearing activity continues to develop until approximately 36 months of age.

Normal Respiratory-Phonatory Development

Birth to Six Months. Because postural control against gravity does not exist initially, active body movement provides the infant with a base from which sounds can be produced on expiration. *Abdominal breathing* is the predominant respiratory pattern, although *asynchronous breathing* may occur during stressful crying, excitement, or effortful activity beginning at birth. The cry modifies in duration, loudness, and intonation as the infant develops active head extension and flexion against gravity, neck elongation, active shoulder girdle depression, spinal extension against gravity, and greater pelvic and hip mobility. The nasal quality of the cry reduces as the oral, pharyngeal, and laryngeal areas enlarge, elongate, and modify in shape, allowing for more active mobility of the soft palate, tongue, hyoid bone, pharyngeal walls, and larynx.

The newborn produces short, low intensity vegetative sounds especially during activities such as feeding. Cooing with nasalized vowel sounds produced with body movements by 2 months of age, modifies to include fricatives, velar consonants, and /m/ by approximately 3 months. There is a significant increase in the types of sounds heard from infants at 4 to 6 months as they begin to produce a greater quantity of throaty sounds in supine, lip sounds in prone, and tongue sounds in sitting.

As teeth begin to erupt at about 6 months, new sounds are made using lip-to-teeth movements. The influence of body position and greater active movements against gravity has become more significant as the child uses vocalization to communicate pleasure or displeasure and to babble during self-initiated play activities.

Seven to Twelve Months. With the development of more active controlled movements against gravity at 7 months, the young child begins to produce sounds separate from body movements. However, there continues to be a general increase in sound production during play which requires active use of the abdominal musculature, active depression of the shoulder girdle with greater scapulo-humeral dissociation, and active spinal mobility. Greater thoracic activity is evident, although abdominal breathing continues to be the predominant breathing pattern.

By 9 months of age, the child produces chains of repeated consonant-vowel combinations composed of bilabial consonants and consonants formed by the use of the front or back of the tongue. These longer sound productions reflect the child's development of more active thoracic and abdominal musculature activity. Asynchronous breathing may still be evident with effort, although the depression noted on inhalation is generally more localized to the sternum.

As the external oblique muscles become more active, and as more controlled, active mobility and stability of the shoulder girdle develops, thoracic expansion increases on inhalation and the abdominals become more active in controlling for longer exhalation. By 13 to 15 months the normal child has developed most of the respiratory control needed for more mature speech production. This is reflected in the child's use of an *abdominal/thoracic breathing* pattern and the production of long chains of consonant-vowel syllables with a wide variety of intonation patterns or jargon during communication.

Prespeech Development in the Infant With Cerebral Palsy

Abnormal Oral-Motor Functioning in Feeding.   In recent years, it has been recognized that a majority of infants diagnosed as cerebral palsied begin with a low postural tone base, or hypotonia. These infants attempt to move with extension as normal infants do, but in order to do so they must use an abnormal quality of extensor activity. Because all movement patterns require a point of stability as well as a point of mobility, the infant with low tone must abnormally hold for stability or fix to attempt movement. This fixing, which occurs initially in proximal parts of the body, will interfere with the infant's ability to develop an active balance of mobility and stability required for all antigravity movements (Bly, 1983).

As the infant continues to move with abnormal muscle tone, fixing, and an abnormal quality of extension, sufficient antigravity flexion cannot be developed. This forces the infant to use compensatory movements which further interfere with the developmental process. Repetition of these abnormal movements, fixations, and compensations creates an abnormal system of sensory-motor feedback on which the infant bases all information about movement and sensation.

As the infant with low postural tone and abnormal extension attempts to lift and turn its head, he or she must fix using the head extensors and extrinsic tongue muscles in order to stabilize. This results in abnormal head/neck hyperextension and *tongue retraction* which is the primary problem for many infants with cerebral palsy, especially those with early feeding problems. As the tongue retracts and the head and neck hyperextend moving the infant's center of gravity posteriorly, the cheeks and lips fall back or retract into gravity, and the jaw depresses and retracts into gravity. Therefore, the infant with an initial problem of tongue retraction and head/neck hyperextension will often reveal some degree of *cheek/lip retraction* and *jaw thrusting with retraction*.

As thin liquids or strained foods are presented to the infant, greater tongue retraction and head/neck hyperextension will occur. In order to control the movement of the liquid or food in the oral cavity, the infant may use compensatory oral movements such as *lip pursing, jaw thrusting with protrusion, jaw clenching, tongue thrusting*, or *excessive tongue protrusion*. Compensatory shoulder elevation occurs to reinforce head and neck stability, especially during swallowing due to the limited mobility and stability of the hyoid.

Functionally, the effects of tongue retraction and head/neck hyperextension on oral-motor functioning in feeding are significant. The infant may have problems initiating suckling or sucking activity. The efficiency of the suckle or suck may be so poor that insufficient nutritional intake results. Poor cheek and lip activity, wide ungraded jaw activity, and limited tongue mobility will result in an excessive loss of liquid and food. Poor coordination of suckling or sucking, swallowing, and breathing may be noted in excessive choking and coughing during all feeding activities.

Another key problem area for infants with cerebral palsy may be seen at the shoulder girdle in the form of abnormal humeral extension/adduction. Active antigravity extension of the thoracic spine does not develop, limiting the infant's ability to develop active stability of the scapulae on the trunk. Therefore, the muscles between the scapula and humerus do not elongate and the upper extremities remain in internal rotation, elbow flexion, forearm pronation, and wrist flexion.

Head/neck hyperextension and tongue retraction are used by this infant in prone to shift weight off of the shoulders in order to view the environment. In sitting, humeral extension/adduction and thoracic flexion will keep these infants' weight so far forward that they must use head/neck hyperextension and tongue retraction to shift their weight posteriorly. However, stronger humeral extension/adduction and abnormal thoracic extension will be used to reinforce head and neck stability, which in turn will shift the weight too far back. These infants are forced to shift their weight forward again by abnormally holding at the positionally shorted rectus abdominus, which pulls downward on the sternum and upward on the pubis, resulting in a posterior pelvic tilt.

Abnormal humeral extension/adduction is generally seen in conjunction with abnormal head/neck hyperextension and tongue retraction. Therefore, infants with early problems at the shoulder girdle also will exhibit the abnormal and compensatory oral-motor functioning and functional consequences of the infant with tongue retraction and head/neck hyperextension.

Infants with low postural tone may not show major movement problems until they need to develop active abdominals, active antigravity thoracic and lumbar spinal extension, and active hip mobility and stability. They may have problems of abnormal lumbar extension with hip flexion, abduction, and external rotation using an excessive frog-leg posture of their lower extremities to fix for stability; or they may use their hip adductors and hamstrings to fix, resulting in abnormal hip extension and adduction.

Although these children may exhibit qualitatively abnormal oral movements early in development, their major problems are most evident in regard to respiratory-phonatory functioning. Poor abdominal and hip activity as well as incomplete development of antigravity spinal extension may result in the use of compensatory humeral extension/adduction, head/neck hyperextension, and tongue retraction. This occurs most often in activities requiring intricate fine-motor coordination. These children, therefore, have the potential for abnormal movements and compensations during oral functioning, which can be seen in the poor coordination of oral movements with swallowing and breathing and in the insufficient development of more intricate dissociated movements of the tongue and jaw.

Abnormal Respiratory-Phonatory Functioning. Neuromotor involvement that restricts or prevents the development of active, coordinated antigravity movements will directly affect respiratory functioning and its coordination with oral activities during feeding, phonation, and sound production. In addition, abnormal musculature activity may prevent the development of anatomical changes necessary for well-coordinated abdominal/thoracic respiratory functioning.

The infant with abnormal tongue retraction, head/neck hyperextension, and humeral extension/adduction may have life-threatening respiratory difficulties from birth. The tongue may be so retracted in the oral cavity that it occludes or greatly limits the size of the oropharynx and nasopharynx, restricting the infant from taking in a sufficient amount of air by nose or mouth. Some infants may attempt to compensate using *tongue retraction with elevation* by pushing the tongue slightly forward while abnormally pushing the front of the tongue up against the hard palate or alveolar ridge. By doing this, the posterior portion of the tongue is brought down, thus opening the nasopharyngeal and oropharyngeal areas for air intake. When crying is produced, it is extremely weak, nasal, irregular, and unsustained.

Abnormal or insufficient development of the head, neck, shoulder girdle, and extrinsic tongue musculature due to abnormal head/neck hyperextension, tongue retraction, and humeral extension/adduction will prevent or restrict development of the balanced musculature activity needed to stabilize the rib cage against the pull of the diaphragm on inhalation. Therefore, asynchronous breathing often becomes this child's predominant respiratory pattern. As shoulder elevation, abnormal holding at a positionally-shorted rectus abdominus, and abnormal oral movements are used for compensation, more severe asynchronous breathing may occur. This will be characterized by excessive lateral flaring of the rib cage, severe retraction of the sternum, and restricted mobility of the diaphragm on inhalation. Immobility and deformities of the rib cage, as well as immobility of the pharyngeal and laryngeal areas, will result.

Functionally, this child will have inadequate coordination of respiration with vocal fold and oral-motor activities. There may be excessive vocal fold adduction (i.e., closed laryngeal blocks) or excessive vocal fold abduction (i.e., open laryngeal blocks) as the child attempts to phonate, allowing only short bursts of sound to be produced. Sound productions will be soft and extremely limited in duration. Hypernasality will occur due to fixation of the tongue musculature which keeps the soft palate in a lowered position. Limited active mobility of the oral, pharyngeal, and laryngeal areas will result in minimal sound and pitch variation.

When a primary problem of abnormal lumbar extension with hip flexion, abduction, and external rotation exists, the hip flexors are maintained in a shortened position, thus pulling the pelvis into an anterior tilt. Since the abdominal musculature cannot actively work in this position to stabilize the lower rib cage, the thoracic area may remain high and barrel-shaped in appearance, and abdominal breathing may be retained as the predominant respiratory pattern. Asynchronous breathing may occur as the child uses compensatory humeral extension/adduction to reinforce spinal extension in prone, sitting, and standing, restricting upper rib cage mobility.

Phonation will be generally weak and breathy. Because abdominal musculature activity is minimal, sound production will be extremely limited in duration. Additional compensations at the head, neck, and oral area may restrict the development of well-coordinated oral-motor and laryngeal functioning for speech.

When there is inadequate development of antigravity thoracic and lumbar extension and insufficient abdominal musculature activity, fixation at the hip adductors and hamstrings may occur. This results in abnormal hip extension/adduction. As children with abnormal hip extension/adduction attempt to function in prone, sitting, and standing, they will use compensatory humeral extension/adduction, abnormal upper trunk flexion, head/neck hyperextension, and abnormal contraction of the rectus abdominus muscle.

The early phonation of a young child with abnormal hip extension/adduction may appear to be within normal limits. However, inadequate development of mobility of the ribs, sternum, and abdominal musculature will occur. Ultimately, this will affect the rate, rhythm, loudness, and duration of the child's extended sound and speech production. Compensatory movements at the head, neck, and shoulder girdle may limit pharyngeal and laryngeal mobility as well as restrict the development of well coordinated fine-motor movements of the oral mechanism required for highly integrated, intelligible speech production.

PRESPEECH AND FEEDING PROGRAMMING

Prespeech and Feeding Assessment

The reader is cautioned that one cannot learn to assess and treat prespeech and feeding problems simply by reading about them. Special training is recommended, to be followed by hands-on experience under the supervision of an experienced professional or as a member of a team which brings together an occupational therapist, physical therapist, speech/language pathologist, and others to share their observations on the influence of positioning and handling on the dynamic functioning of respiratory, laryngeal, pharyngeal, and oral mechanisms.

A comprehensive prespeech assessment is conducted to obtain information on the movements of the individual parts of the child's oral mechanism during feeding and sound production; the quality and coordination of these oral movements; the influence of postural tone, movement, and sensory stimulation on oral-motor and respiratory-phonatory functioning; the coordination of respiration with feeding and sound production; and the child's use of communication (e.g., facial expression, gestures, eye pointing, sound production) during movement and feeding activities. This information is gathered through careful questioning of the caregiver, observation of the child with the caregiver during prespeech activities, and direct testing by the evaluator.

A thorough observation of the child's movement patterns, postural tone, and responses to different sensory stimulation is essential. Abnormal or compensatory activity at the head, neck, shoulder girdle, trunk, pelvis, and hips must be examined in regard to its effect on oral-motor and respiratory-phonatory functioning. In addition, oral and respiratory functioning in feeding, communication, and sound production activities must be observed in regard to their effects on changes in postural tone and general movement. These observations cannot be generalized from evaluations done for other purposes, but must be made as part of the prespeech assessment because of the intricate relationship between movement, sensory-motor feedback, and prespeech functioning.

Analysis of the child's feeding activity comprises a significant part of the prespeech assessment. The caregiver should be asked to describe nutritional intake, mealtime length, preferred food textures, feeding utensils used, and positioning used for mealtime feeding. Specifics about the child's movements during feeding activities should also be ascertained. Special care must be taken not to require the caregiver to make qualitative judgments on the child's feeding activity or to make a decision concerning the existence of a feeding problem. Such a decision by the caregiver will be based on the amount of nutritional intake and not on the quality of oral musculature activity, which is the evaluator's primary purpose for investigating this aspect of prespeech functioning.

Observation of interactions between caregiver and child as well as the procedures used by the caregiver during the feeding process is extremely important. The evaluator should place special emphasis on obtaining information which describes the initial position of the child and any changes in position that may occur; any modifications that have been made in feeding utensils (e.g., enlarged nipple hole); how the caregiver presents the food or liquid and the child's response to this presentation; the jaw, cheek, lip, and tongue movements used by the child as well as any changes in these movements that may occur; the child's coordination of breathing with oral movements for feeding; the ways that the child communicates and interacts with the caregiver; and the caregiver's response to and interpretation of the child's interactions.

After observing the child and caregiver, the evaluator may decide that direct testing is required to analyze previously observed movements and to attempt to modify oral-motor and respiratory-phonatory functioning through changes in positioning, handling, food textures, or food presentation. Opportunities may be provided for the child to experience feeding activities that have not been previously attempted or were unsuccessful in the past (e.g., presenting liquid by cup or a bottle to a breastfed infant over 6 months of age; placing a cracker on the side gums of an infant over 5 months of age). The evaluator may provide handling which facilitates more active postural control and movement against gravity in order to stimulate changes in the child's respiratory-phonatory coordination, sound production, and general communication activities. Through direct testing, the evaluator not only analyzes the child's present, observable level of functioning, but also attempts to modify sensory and motor input in order to obtain information which suggests the child's potential for future prespeech development.

Most commercially available evaluation tools attempt to look at prespeech functioning using a more general, milestone approach. *The Pre-Speech Assessment Scale* (Morris, 1982b) is the only evaluation tool now available which provides a format with guidelines and scoring procedures for the assessment of normal and abnormal components of prespeech functioning during the first 2 years. However, whether formal or informal testing procedures are used, the evaluator must have an extensive base of knowledge in all components of normal and abnormal prespeech development if assessment information is to be properly obtained and interpreted in regard to the development of appropriate intervention programming.

Prespeech and Feeding Intervention

Intervention Strategies. An appropriate prespeech and feeding intervention program is developed by the speech-language pathologist with input from all intervention team members. It must incorporate intervention strategies which emphasizes the child's need to develop controlled musculature activity for oral-motor, respiratory-phonatory, and communication functioning through direct treatment as well as those which emphasize modifications of the child's mealtime feeding for increased nutritional intake.

Generally, it is advisable to address, initially, problems of limited nutritional intake during mealtime feeding in order to reduce parental anxieties and major medical concerns. Often, modifications can be made in the child's positioning for feeding, the types of food and liquid textures being given, the utensils used for feeding, and the ways in which the food and liquid are presented in order to make feeding more successful. When food intake is not substantially increased through these modifications or when there are major medically related concerns (e.g., dehydration, aspiration, failure to thrive) requiring immediate increases in nutritional intake to avoid life-threatening situations, it may be necessary to recommend other procedures such as tube feeding which will increase the child's food intake while reducing parental fears and medical complications. It should be evident that procedures directed toward mealtime feeding are being implemented for the sole purpose of increasing the amount of food and liquid that the child receives. Therefore, functional prespeech and feeding treatment goals which must emphasize the development of active components of oral-motor, respiratory-phonatory, and communication functioning cannot be expected to take precedence during mealtime feeding activities.

The intervention strategies implemented by the speech-language pathologist during direct, hands-on treatment must reflect the relationship between general antigravity movement development and the development of functional prespeech movement components. This emphasis on the development of functional prespeech components can only be stimulated through handling that encourages the child's active use of musculature in a variety of sensory-motor experiences.

The development of well-coordinated oral-motor, respiratory-phonatory, speech, and communication functioning takes time. As new movement components develop and are carried over into daily activities such as mealtime feeding, they become active parts of the child's general functioning abilities. Therefore, prespeech and feeding intervention programming must incorporate strategies which recognize the intricate connections between the development of the components of prespeech functioning through direct treatment and the carry-over of these developmental components into daily maintenance activities such as feeding at mealtime.

Handling and Positioning for Prespeech Functioning. The terms "handling" and "positioning" are often used interchangeably, incorrectly suggesting that they represent equivalent treatment concepts. This has resulted in an excessive emphasis on proper positioning rather than on active handling as a basis for active prespeech functioning. Handling and positioning are both significant aspects of prespeech intervention, but they must be recognized as two distinct concepts.

According to Bergen and Colangelo (1982), "proper positioning and adapted equipment provide a necessary adjunct to therapy, carrying over goals into all areas of daily living (home, school, work, etc.), normalizing tone, and facilitating more normal movement" (p. 3). Proper positioning can reduce the influence of abnormal movements, decrease the potential for deformities, and create a base of central stability which allows for more functional fine motor control.

In prespeech intervention, proper positioning provides a base of good body alignment for better oral-motor, respiratory-phonatory, and sensory-motor functioning during carry-over activities such as mealtime feeding (Alexander, 1983; Alexander & Bigge, 1962; Bergen & Colangelo, 1982; Connor, Williamson, & Siepp, 1978; Finnie, 1975; Morris, 1977, 1982a; Mueller, 1975a; Sâlék, 1983; Scherzer & Tscharnuter, 1982). This base of good body alignment is characterized by neck elongation with neutral head flexion; symmetrical and stable shoulder girdle depression with scapulo-humeral dissociation; symmetrical trunk elongation; neutral positioning of a stable, symmetrical pelvis; hip stability with neutral abduction and rotation; and symmetrical, stable positioning of the feet flat on a surface. If proper positioning with good body alignment is not achieved due to severe physical deformity or improper equipment adaptation, functional fine motor control during mealtime feeding cannot be expected.

Because the central stability obtained through proper positioning is static, it does not stimulate the development of coordinated, antigravity musculature activity in response to weight shift which is required if fine motor control is to be integrated into all elements of a child's functional movement. The development of well coordinated oral-motor and respiratory-phonatory functioning produced by the child's active use of musculature is stimulated in prespeech treatment which incorporates dynamic handling through movement rather than static positioning.

Handling which combines the inhibition of abnormal movement patterns and the facilitation of more normal movement patterns (Bobath & Bobath, 1964) is most often discussed in regard to physical therapy with goals for the development of righting and equilibrium reactions. Although the general handling techniques used in prespeech treatment may appear similar to those used in other treatment modalities, the ultimate functional goals and objectives will relate directly to the components of prespeech functioning (e.g., rib cage mobility and stability; coordination of breathing with sound production; active lip closure; forward/back, up/down, and lateral tongue movements; graded jaw movements) that the individual child needs to develop (Alexander, 1983; Connor et al., 1978; Mueller, 1975b; Scherzer & Tscharnuter, 1982).

Modifying Oral Tactile Sensitivity.   Oral tactile hypersensitivity or hyposensitivity will have a direct negative effect on a child's oral-motor functioning. Therefore, it is necessary to incorporate activities into a child's prespeech intervention program which help to modify responses to oral tactile stimulation (Alexander, 1983; Morris, 1977, 1978, 1982a; Mueller, 1972).

Infants with abnormal postural tone and movement develop a base of abnormal sensory-motor feedback which directly affects their responses to tactile input throughout the body, while also placing restrictions on their sensory-motor experiences. This requires that programming initially emphasize incorporating handling to stimulate more normal postural tone and movement with presentation of well graded tactile stimulation. As more normal responses to tactile input occur throughout the body, emphasis can be directed toward modifying sensitivity to tactile stimulation at the face and in the oral area.

The infant or child will generally have more difficulty tolerating light touch and poorly graded, quickly presented tactile stimulation. Firm rubbing and stroking of the body, face, and oral area will be better tolerated. The speed of presentation must be carefully graded since the hypersensitive child may initially respond more positively to slow, graded tactile input, while the hyposensitive child may require a more rapid speed of well graded stimulation.

It is important that oral tactile stimulation activities be carried over by the caregiver. Firm rubbing and stroking of the infant's body and face with a washcloth, squeeze toys, or the baby's own hands should be incor-

porated along with graded handling and proper positioning into play activities at home. Early, consistent presentation of deep pressure oral tactile
input directed toward the gums, teeth, tongue, and hard palate using a
small toothbrush presented during play or feeding activities can stimulate more normal responses to touch in the mouth while reducing the
potential for *tonic biting*. Cleaning a child's face with a soft, damp washcloth using well graded, slow, deep pressure rather than a quick, light touch
can provide good tactile stimulation to the face as well as to the gums and
inner surfaces of the cheeks and lips.

Oral-motor functioning for feeding, sound play, and speech is directly
influenced by the oral tactile sensory feedback the child receives. If well
graded experiences with oral tactile input are not provided, the child's
potential for more normal oral movements will be greatly reduced.

Modifying Oral-Motor Functioning for Feeding   Once a base of more
central body control has been introduced through handling during treatment and proper positioning during mealtime feeding, attention can be
directed toward presenting stimulation for more specific oral-motor functioning changes. The most significant modifications can be made in oral
movements during feeding activities through changes in food textures,
choice of feeding utensils, and food presentation (Alexander, 1983; Morris,
1978, 1982a; Pipes, 1981; Scherzer & Tscharnuter, 1982).

Generally, thin liquids and strained, pureed foods are the most difficult for children with neuromotor involvement to handle. Thickened foods
and liquids provide greater sensory information to the child and are
usually more easily controlled.

More efficient sucking and swallowing activity can be stimulated
through the use of thicker liquids such as fruit nectars and thicker foods
such as ground table foods. Thin liquids such as juice or milk can be
thickened by adding foods such as baby cereal or applesauce. Strained
foods can be mixed with wheat germ, cracker crumbs, or cereal to create
a thickened consistency.

The early introduction of solid foods (5–6 months of age) is extremely
important for the stimulation of more normal oral tactile sensitivity and
for the development of chewing and biting. Generally, soft solids such as
crackers or cheese are the easiest to start with since they can be broken
up by early munching activity and mix well with saliva for easy swallowing. Formed solids such as grapes or raisins are more difficult because they
require that the child have coordinated chewing and grinding movements
as well as the ability to control two separate textures in the mouth—the
saliva, and the formed solid.

Changing the type of nipple used in bottledrinking may help an infant
to produce a more efficient sucking or suckling pattern. If the nipple hole
is so enlarged that the formula or milk flows too rapidly into the infant's

mouth, abnormal sucking and swallowing activity will probably result. A short nipple may not provide enough surface for the infant to obtain sufficient closure for active sucking. A variety of nipples should be tried to see if changes in the shape, size, or texture of the nipple will stimulate more active oral movements. If sucking continues to be poor or severe tonic bite activity exists, the presentation of thickened liquids by spoon or cup may be introduced.

It is important to choose a spoon which fits within the child's mouth without touching the side gums or teeth. The spoon should be blunt and have a shallow bowl so that minimal lip activity is required for food removal. Brittle plastic spoons and plastic-coated spoons should not be used with children who tonic bite. If the child is orally hypersensitive, a less stimulating utensil such as a tongue depressor may be used to present thickened food.

When introducing liquid intake by cup, it is generally better to use a flexible plastic cup with a small rim which will not interfere with attempts at lip closure. A section of the top of the cup may be cut out so that liquid can be directed to the mouth without the child's head pushing back into hyperextension.

The positive effects of proper positioning or handling and the appropriate use of food textures and utensils can be eliminated if the presentation of the food and liquid is overstimulating for the child. The feeder should be positioned at, or slightly below, the child's eye level in order to avoid stimulating abnormal head and neck hyperextension. Feeding utensils should be presented and removed at, or slightly below, the level of the child's mouth in a graded manner so that the visual stimulation does not elicit abnormal activity.

Active handling, proper positioning, the stimulation of more normal oral tactile sensitivity, the modification of food and liquid textures, the use of appropriate feeding utensils, and the grading of food presentation are essential to prespeech and feeding intervention programming. However, the suggestions provided in all of these areas will only be effective if appropriate for the individual child.

Comprehensive prespeech and feeding intervention programming is not only concerned with a child's ability to eat. Its goals and objectives must reflect the specific active movement components required for oral-motor, respiratory-phonatory, sound production, and communication functioning. When the components of the normal developmental process are truly understood, the significance of the relationship between prespeech and feeding development and overall speech-language development, especially in regard to the special needs of the child with cerebral palsy, should be clear.

DEFINITIONS

Terms Related to Normal Oral-Motor and Respiratory Functioning

Abdominal Breathing Belly breathing pattern with active lowering of the diaphragm and expansion of the abdominal area on inspiration.

Abdominal/Thoracic Breathing Breathing pattern with active elevation of the rib cage and lowering of the diaphragm on inspiration, and active use of the abdominals to control expiration.

Asynchronous Breathing Breathing pattern with strong contraction of the diaphragm, expansion of the abdominal area, and depression of the thoracic cavity and/or sternum on inspiration; occurs with effort or stress in infants who have not yet developed active antigravity trunk control.

Automatic Phasic Bite-Release Pattern Response to tactile input on the biting surfaces of the gums or teeth composed of small, rhythmical up/down jaw movements; occurs until about 5 months of age.

Chewing Process used to break up solids with lateral, spreading, and rolling movements of the tongue propelling the food between the teeth, and rotary movements of the jaw.

Controlled, Sustained Bite Easy, graded closure of the teeth through the food with an easy release for chewing; seen at about 12 months of age.

Gag Response Response to tactile input on the back of the tongue or pharyngeal area composed of jaw extension, forward/downward tongue movement, and pharyngeal constriction with head and neck extension; strong at birth, reducing in strength by 7 months; still evident through adulthood.

Jaw Stabilization Active, internal jaw control with minimal jaw movement used in cupdrinking; initially obtained by biting on the cup rim at about 15 months of age; gradually develops using active jaw musculature by 24 months of age.

Munching Early chewing pattern composed of rhythmical up/down jaw movements with spreading, flattening, and some up/down tongue movements; begins at about 5 months of age with the introduction of solids.

Rooting Response Response to tactile input on the lips or cheeks characterized by mouth opening and head turning in the direction of the touch; occurs until about 4 to 5 months of age.

Rotary Jaw Movements Activity used in chewing which increases from 15 to 36 months of age reflecting the integration of up/down, forward/backward, lateral, diagonal, circular-diagonal, diagonal-rotary, and circular-rotary jaw movements.

Sucking A rhythmical method for obtaining liquid or food characterized by the active coordination of small up/down jaw movements, up/down tongue body movements, lip approximation, and cheek activity; negative pressure is built up in the oral cavity due to the more closed mouth position.

Suckling   An early lick-type of sucking pattern composed of rhythmical forward/backward tongue movements, large rhythmical up/down jaw movements, and minimal lip and cheek activity.

Tongue Lateralization   Active movement of the tongue to the sides of the mouth to maintain and propel food between the biting surfaces during the chewing process; begins at 6 to 7 months with horizontal shifts or gross rolling movements of the tongue.

Terms Related to Abnormal Oral Functioning

Cheek/Lip Retraction   Abnormal pulling back of the cheeks and lips for abnormal stabilization; the lips appear thin, forming a tight line across the mouth; initially seen in conjunction with abnormal head/neck hyperextension and tongue retraction.

Jaw Clenching   Abnormal jaw closure which occurs as a compensation for excessive jaw instability; the jaw is unstable so that graded, controlled jaw elevation cannot occur.

Jaw Thrusting   Abnormally strong depression of the lower jaw; the extent and force of the lower jaw depression is greater than that seen in normal suckling; the jaw may become stuck in an open position; reinforces abnormal head/neck hyperextension.

Jaw Thrusting with Protrusion   Abnormally strong depression with forward pushing of the lower jaw; often seen initially as attempts are made to close an unstable jaw which has been opened with thrusting and retraction; occurs as a compensatory jaw movement.

Jaw Thrusting with Retraction   Abnormally strong depression with backward movement of the lower jaw; initially seen in conjunction with abnormal head/neck hyperextension and tongue retraction.

Lip Pursing   Purse-string positioning of the lips and cheeks; the cheeks and lip corners are slightly retracted for abnormal stability while the central portion of the lips are semi-protruded and appear to be puckering.

Tongue Retraction   Abnormal stabilization of the tongue back in the oral cavity; the posterior portion of the tongue may appear humped up in the back of the oral cavity; the tongue is thick in appearance; reinforces abnormal head/neck hypertension.

Tongue Retraction with Elevation   Abnormal stabilization of the tongue back in the oral cavity with the front of the tongue elevated, pushing up against the alveolar ridge; the back of the tongue is lowered due to the anterior tongue elevation; generally occurs as a compensation for excessive tongue instability.

Tongue Thrusting   Abnormally strong forward pushing of the tongue which is bunched and thick in contour; generally occurs as a compensatory tongue movement.

Tonic Biting   Abnormally strong jaw closure in response to tactile stimulation on the biting surfaces of the gums or teeth; stronger jaw closure with increased abnormal head, neck, and trunk extension occurs with attempts to remove the stimulation; the jaw is stuck in a closed position.

REFERENCES

Alexander, R. (1983). Developing pre-speech and feeding abilities in children. In S. Shanks (Ed.), *Nursing and the management of pediatric communication disorders.* San Diego, CA: College-Hill Press.

Alexander, R., & Bigge, J. (1982). Facilitation of language and speech. In J. Bigge (Ed.), *Teaching individuals with physical and multiple disabilities* (pp. 257–289). Columbus, OH: Charles E. Merrill.

Bergen, A., & Colangelo, C. (1982). *Positioning the client with central nervous system deficits: The wheelchair and other adapted equipment.* New York: Valhalla Rehabilitation Publications.

Bly, L. (1983). *The components of normal movement during the first year of life and abnormal motor development.* Chicago: Neuro-Developmental Treatment Association.

Bobath, K., & Bobath, B. (1964). The facilitation of normal postural reactions and movements in the treatment of cerebral palsy. *Physiotherapy, 50,* 246–262.

Bosma, J. (Ed.). (1972). *Third symposium on oral-sensation and perception.* Springfield, IL: Charles C Thomas.

Bosma, J. (1978). Structure and function of the infant oral and pharyngeal mechanisms. In J. Wilson (Ed.), *Oral-Motor function and dysfunction in children* (pp. 33–78). Chapel Hill: University of North Carolina.

Connor, F., Williamson, G., & Siepp, J. (Eds.). (1978). *Program guide for infants and toddlers with neuromotor and other developmental disabilities.* New York: Teachers College Press.

Finnie, N. (1975). *Handling the young cerebral palsied child at home.* New York: E. P. Dutton.

Morris, S. (1977). *Program guidelines for children with feeding problems.* Edison, NJ: Childcraft.

Morris, S. (1978). Treatment of children with oral-motor dysfunction. In J. Wilson (Ed.), *Oral-Motor function and dysfunction in children* (pp. 163–193). Chapel Hill: University of North Carolina.

Morris, S. (1982a). *The normal acquisition of oral feeding skills: Implications for assessment and treatment.* New York: Therapeutic Media.

Morris, S. (1982b). *Pre-Speech assessment scale.* Clifton, NJ: J. A. Preston.

Mueller, H. (1972). Facilitating feeding and pre-speech. In P. Pearson & C. Williams (Eds.), *Physical therapy services in the development disabilities* (pp. 113–132). Springfield, IL: Charles C Thomas.

Mueller, H. (1975a). Feeding. In N. Finnie (Ed.), *Handling the young cerebral palsied child at home* (pp. 113–132). New York: E. P. Dutton.

Mueller, H. (1975b). Speech. N. Finnie (Ed.), *Handling the young cerebral palsied child at home* (pp. 133–140). New York: E. P. Dutton.

Peiper, A. (1963). *Cerebral function in infancy and childhood.* New York: Consultant Bureau.

Pipes, P. (1981). *Nutrition in infancy and childhood* (2nd ed.). St. Louis: C. V. Mosby.

Sálék, B. (1983). Principles of therapeutic positioning in infants and young children. In M. Braun & M. Palmer (Eds.), *Early detection and treatment of the infant and young child with neuromuscular disorders* (pp. 77–119). New York: Therapeutic Media.

Scherzer, A., & Tscharnuter, I. (1982). *Early diagnosis and therapy in cerebral palsy.* New York: Marcel Dekker.

CHAPTER 8

Handling, Positioning, and Adaptive Equipment

Jacqueline M. Doherty

Doherty maintains that abnormal positions assumed during improper handling, or when lying or sitting, interfere with neuromuscular development and aggravate the child's neuromuscular dysfunction. Positions may be produced by proper handling and positioning which facilitate development of motor control for feeding, communicating, and classroom activities. For many persons with cerebral palsy, adaptive equipment is necessary to aid in carrying out the activities of daily living.

1. *It is essential that parents and all rehabilitation team members understand the need for, and proper techniques of, handling and positioning cerebral palsied children. As you read this chapter, make a list of techniques of handling and positioning the speech/language pathologist should learn and note when they should be used.*

2. *How a cerebral palsied child is seated influences speech production and the use of communication aids. What factors should the speech/language pathologist consider when staff members are planning seating for a severely involved child or evaluating the adequacy of a child's seating?*

3. *Assume that your caseload includes several severely involved school age cerebral palsied clients. What equipment would you want for positioning, and how and when would you use it? (Review this question after reading Chapter 9.)*

INTRODUCTION

During the first months after birth, unless they are held, infants lie in either a prone or supine position unable to support themselves in other positions. As they are held, bounced, bathed, fed, and generally moved about by the caretaker, stimulation received by all the senses is fed into the central nervous system which develops and learns, practices, and remembers. When lying on their backs, infants may assume a "frog" position (Figure 8.1). The asymmetrical tonic neck position (flexion of arm and leg on same side of body, with head turned toward extended extremities) and other infantile positions are often observed, but normally developing infants are able to move in and out of these with ease.

Infants systematically acquire the strength and neuromuscular control needed to roll, sit, crawl, stand, walk, and eventually run, skip, and jump. By the end of their first 6 months, most infants can maintain sitting posture, which allows free movement of the arms and hands to manipulate objects. They learn to counter gravitational forces, first from the broad base of round sitting (knees flexed toward sides with soles together). Gradually they learn to adjust to gravity with bases of decreasing size. From a four-point support (hands and knees) they move to a crawling position. From a standing base of two flat feet, they progress to walking where weight is momentarily balanced on part of one foot. Neuromuscular control now enables the child to maintain balance even when moving. Most infants progress through the various stages of acquiring body control and locomotion without special attention.

Unfortunately, this is not so for many children with cerebral palsy. As a result of their brain pathology, they may remain dependent on low-level reflex activity, locked into positions because of spasticity or relegated to uncontrolled motion. Unless performed correctly, handling for play, bathing, and feeding may aggravate the condition. Sitting without support may be unattainable, and improper seating may interfere with development and function. No lasting effect is achieved through the treatment if most of the child's time is spent lying on the back with the arms extended and rotated outward in abnormal posture, or seated with the trunk slouched and neck flexed on the chest, or being fed with the head back and food poured down the throat. For children with neuromuscular dysfunction, most aspects of their lives must be carefully managed.

LIVING MANAGEMENT

It is essential that all individuals involved in family life, care, and recreation, as well as those involved in treatment and education, learn and practice the principles of good handling and use of appropriate equipment which will stimulate the central nervous system.

Need for an Integrated Approach

In earlier programs for managing cerebral palsy, each discipline developed its own program with little interaction among the individual disciplines. Today it is recognized that therapists, parents, and other professional workers must cooperate in evaluation, planning, and carrying out a program.

This approach requires that all disciplines have an understanding of problems that earlier were not considered in their area of expertise. For example, educators must be aware how moving children out of their chairs into other appropriate positions will facilitate the educational process (Bobath, 1972). Speech/language pathologists need a basic understanding of posture and gross motor activities in order to promote vocalization and to help the child use communication aids. Physical and occupational therapists need an understanding of basic communication processes and education programs in order to devise the best seating for the classroom and optimal positioning for communication training.

Staff Training

If we, as professionals, expect families to appreciate the importance of total living management, we must demonstrate a total living-therapy-education program. It is important to begin with an evaluation involving all therapists and teachers. The program will then develop as a group effort and will grow and change as the needs of the child change.

When children are enrolled in a school, whether it be day or residential, the same importance should be given to total care. While therapists have an ongoing responsibility to supervise handling, positioning, and the use of equipment in the school, dormitory, dining, and recreational areas, all persons who work with the child are responsible for carrying out the total program.

Inservice training sessions conducted on a regular basis are essential to impart information to professional and nonprofessional staff. These communication sessions are usually more effective when conducted in a problem solving form rather than as lectures or in a "how to" approach. Not only do these sessions provide education for the staff, they also develop rapport among the staff. Refresher sessions for experienced staff members are needed, as well as orientation sessions for the new staff. Reference material such as *Handling the Young Cerebral Palsy Child at Home* (Finnie, 1970) should be readily available. Large charts with drawings, illustrating proper and improper use of equipment may be displayed in various areas of the building. Photographs showing familiar staff members and children often arouse more interest than charts and drawings.

In nonresidential settings, a close relationship with the family must be established and maintained to create this total program. A home visit by a staff member may result in greater insight into the child's general lifestyle. Conferences in which family members have the opportunity to observe and participate with the educator and therapist promote understanding of the child's problems and effective methods of dealing with these problems.

HANDLING

The first concern should be with the correct way to pick up and carry a child with cerebral palsy. The most natural instinct of the average person is to reach under the child's arms and lift the child with legs extended to the caretaker's shoulder. This is fine for the normal child who can readily move, but handling the handicapped child in this manner continues to feed into the central nervous system sensations of abnormal posturing. A child must be lifted and held in a way that will reverse the abnormal posturing and promote a good body alignment, giving support only where needed.

The child who lies in the "frog" position (Figure 8.1) would have better sensory input if held in a flexed position (Figure 8.2) with the legs brought forward to the midline of the body. Holding a child in this flexed position makes it easier to place him or her in a chair. The hips are flexed to a 90° angle and are easily put well back into the seat when attaching the hip control strap. If bending the hips is difficult due to extensor thrusting of the body, placing the child in a side-lying position for a few minutes will reflexively reduce the extension (Figure 8.3).

The child whose shoulder position prevents the arms and hands from coming forward and being seen or touching will never have the opportunity to learn from tactile stimulation and manipulation. Holding the child in a position with the shoulders rotated forward, thus allowing some hand contact, may give impetus to the learning process. The child's hands should be kept in the most functional position possible to promote maximum use.

Awareness of abnormal postures and the methods of controlling them with our own bodies or special apparatus is more effective when extended to all activities of daily living. Dressing, bathing, or just playing provides opportunities for counteracting abnormal processes.

LYING

Children need to be on the floor at times but here, too, concern for good positioning is essential.

Side-Lying

The side-lyer is a useful and easily constructed piece of equipment. When placed on the floor in a side-lyer, the child may interact with other chil-

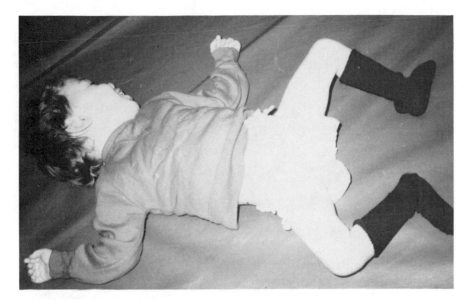

Figure 8.1.   Frog position.

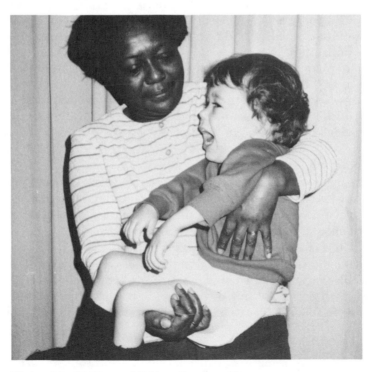

Figure 8.2.   Holding a child in a flexed position.

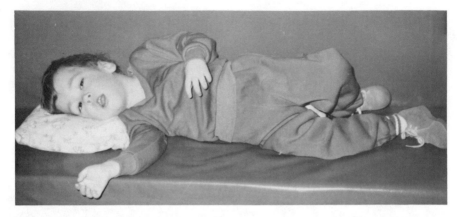

Figure 8.3. Side-lying position.

dren while being supported for correct body alignment. This position facilitates bringing the hands toward midline where they can more easily be viewed and where they can possibly contact each other (Figure 8.3). The side-lying position is also indicated for children who have a diagnosis of scoliosis (curvature of the spine). The side position aligns the trunk when lying on the concave side. Additional opportunities for using this side position are at nap or bedtime, when bed rails and pillows are used for support and stabilization.

Construction of a side-lyer is uncomplicated. Materials needed include two 5' x 12" x 3/4" x 1" thick boards, 1-inch foam, and vinyl. The two 12-inch-wide boards are attached at a right angle; each board is padded with 1-inch foam and covered with vinyl. The body is controlled either by a padded block placed in front of the trunk or by wide straps.

Prone-Lying

Foam rubber wedges are positioning aids for prone-lying. The height of the wedge is selected to permit a comfortable elbow support position, or easy arm extension. Only when the child has some shoulder and head control should prone-lying be used (Figure 8.4).

The use of wedges is indicated for the child who has hip and knee flexion tendencies. When lying prone on a wedge, gravity works to extend the whole body, with the lower extremities kept in alignment by sandbags placed on either side of the legs. When a cerebral palsied child assumes an abnormally extended posture, this position should not be used.

Semi-Lying

When a child needs more control or support over the entire body to maintain alignment due to abnormal posturing, a large bean bag is useful.

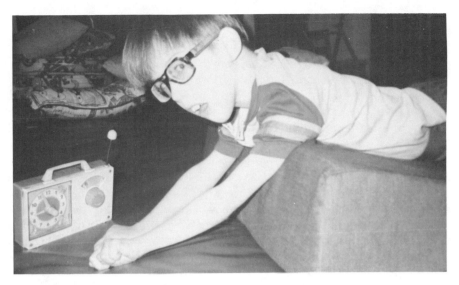

Figure 8.4. Prone-lying position.

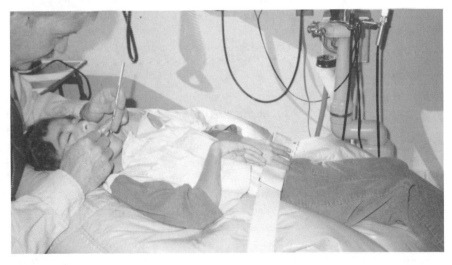

Figure 8.5. Semi-lying position.

A bean bag offers support for the child when lying between a supine and an upright position; however, frequent monitoring is necessary because the beans tend to shift with body movement and the support can be lost or improperly placed. At the Home of the Merciful Saviour, bean bags have been used in the dental program (Figure 8.5). When used in the dental chair, they give a small child comfort and security. Most dental chairs rarely fit small and poorly controlled bodies.

THE UPRIGHT POSITION

Ability to sit upright is important for physical, cognitive, and social-emotional development. Hulme, Poor, Schulein, and Pezzino (1983) note that appropriate seating facilitates development of arm and hand skills, results in caretakers spending more time with clients, and generally aids in carrying out training programs. They suggest that development of communication and subsequent learning often depend on this ability.

Learning progresses in proportion to the amount and variety of sensory input and the ability to process this stimulation. Prior to attaining the upright sitting position, the visual environment of the infant is limited as are opportunities for tactile stimulation (Figure 8.6). In the upright position, the head and eyes may be moved for wide examination of the environs, and eye-hand coordination progresses as the child observes manual activity (Figure 8.7). Tactile stimulation occurs as the hands are brought together at midline and a constantly growing number of objects are manipulated and felt.

The upright position encourages and facilitates interaction with people and objects, thus contributing to development of self-awareness and differentiation of self from others. The intellectual abilities of children who cannot maintain head and trunk control are often underestimated, and these children may even be avoided because of their grotesque posture.

Considerations for Good Seating

Equipment providing acceptable seating for handicapped individuals is an important treatment modality. Among the various types of seating, wheelchairs are especially important because they provide both support and mobility. They should not be considered as a last resort in handling the severely handicapped person, but rather as a beginning step in the creation of an environment to make life more meaningful.

Comfort. A favorite chair may be comfortable, not necessarily for its softness, but for the support given in relationship to the particular activity in which the person is involved. A soft sofa may be appropriate for watching TV, even when one sits in a slouched position. But, when typing or writing, hip and trunk stability is needed to give freedom for arm use. People with normal body tone are able to bridge this gap, but the severely handicapped individual constantly needs support and assistance to reduce strain and ensure comfort and maximum function.

Safety. Wheelchairs should be designed or modified with the security of the user in mind. No wheelchair should be used without a working pair of brakes that are checked regularly. Inefficient brakes are dangerous to those placing the child in the chair, as well as to the child riding in it. No one should be removed or placed in a wheelchair without first determining that the brakes are locked.

Safety belts with a secure buckle attachment are needed on all wheelchairs. If one is not already attached to the chair at the time of purchase, a strap should be secured into the seat before using the chair.

Suitability.   Size, height, weight, and ease of movement determine the suitability of the wheelchair. Special adaptations may be used in a chair to meet specific needs, but it is important to start with a chair of the correct size. Projection for future growth must be considered, but should not be an overriding factor in selecting a chair.

Proper height from the floor may mean that the child will be able to join the family at the dinner table. It may also mean the opportunity to participate in group activities in the classroom. Although no wheelchair is easy to lift, some are lighter than others. When chairs are too heavy to be placed in the trunk of a car, outside excursions may be reduced to only essential trips. However, sturdiness should not be sacrificed for lightness. Caster size affects mobility. Chairs with small casters will move easily on flat, smooth surfaces, but will be difficult to move on thick pile carpeting.

Cost.   Because any wheelchair is an expensive item, comparison shopping is advised. Generally, it is advisable to order a basic chair without costly adaptations, if adjustments and adaptations can be made by parents and/or therapists.

Convenience.   When a substantial amount of time is spent taking the chair apart and putting it back together before it can be used, transportation of the person and the chair may be minimized.

Adapting Wheelchairs

Special seating and seat positioning have been used in the management of cerebral palsy children for many years. The wooden "relaxation chair" was an early attempt to provide comfortable, controlled seating for the severely involved child. It was more successfully used in schools where floors were smooth and its small wheels did not unduly hamper maneuverability. The relaxation chair had many disadvantages, however. The child's body rested against a tilted back, making the plane of vision too high to enable the child to enjoy interaction with classmates. Feeding the child was easier, but normal oral activity was lacking. Seating was a containment rather than an extension of therapy.

When principles of normal growth and development became the bases for therapeutic procedures, the need for trunk control and stability, and the importance of automatic reflex activity were recognized. This led to the revaluation of seating practices, and more appropriate approaches to positioning the disabled individual were developed (Letts, 1983).

Physical and occupational therapists, with their knowledge of gross motor function, are primarily involved in the adaptation of wheelchairs, but neither can operate efficiently without the help of all those involved in education, therapy, recreation, and general care. The determination of a successful seating arrangement is based on good posture and maximum function in all environments over an extended period of time.

The standard wheelchair has a seat and back of vinyl that bows with the body weight, providing very little, if any, support to maintain the upright position or provide stability at the hips.

"Where do I start" is a frequently asked question. The answer is "from the bottom up," as a stable hip position is the basis for trunk and head control. Sitting with the hips at a 90° angle is the most natural position, but sometimes the front of the solid seat must be raised to counteract stiffening and extension of the body and to provide comfortable and controlled posture (Hildreth, Horsman, & Slurtevante, 1982).

The Seat.   The seat is made from a board 3/4 inch thick cut to fit snugly in the seat resting on the solid side supports of the wheelchair. The chair must always provide an even base that extends from the hips forward to the bend of the knee without causing the lower leg to extend. When there is a leg length discrepancy, both thighs will have equal support if the seat is cut to accommodate the position.

For comfort, all wooden inserts need 1-inch sponge padding and vinyl upholstery.

The Back.   To facilitate back extension, a solid padded board, similar to the seat board, is put in place between the uprights of the chair. The firm back reduces the possibility of sitting with the spine in a "C" curve position. When head control is lacking, the back should be high enough to offer optimal support. Straps or ties attached to the top of the back board can be tied around the push handles to prevent the board from dropping. The forward position of the back board determines the depth of the seat, which should be a consideration during construction. Seats and backs may be attached when more stability is needed or side pieces are to be added. When this is done, however, the entire insert becomes somewhat more difficult to remove from the chair.

Wedges.   Leg positions or leg movement cause seating problems even when the hips and trunk are in a controlled position. When knees are unable to stay apart, a well padded wooden wedge is placed in the seat between the legs, extending from the knee to above mid thigh. The size of the wedge is determined by the space needed to keep the legs in alignment and should be high enough to prevent the legs from riding over it. Wedges are used only to keep the knees apart and should never be used to force the body back into the chair.

When the thighs spread too far apart, long blocks of wood are attached to the seat on the outer side of the legs to provide symmetry.

Footplates.   To keep feet from dropping and heel cords from tightening, a 90° angle resting position should be used. For the child who thrusts his or her body out of the chair, footplates are adjustable and may be raised when it is deemed advisable to have an increased angle for the hips and knees.

Safety Belts. A strong seat belt is essential for safety and control of hip position. When hip control is needed, the strap should angle forward from the junction of the back and seat, attached to the wheelchair by the screws that hold the seat to the frame. This position places the strap over the pelvis rather than around the waist or over the legs where a child can easily wiggle out of position.

If the wheelchair is not equipped with a seat belt, or if the seat belt is improperly placed, new seat belts can be made from heavy cotton webbing using prong buckles, or auto seat belts may be attached.

Trays. When properly constructed and fitted, trays that rest on the arms of wheelchairs are valuable in many ways. They provide a resting place for elbows, which in turn gives support to the shoulders and head. They provide the wheelchair-bound child with a surface for eating, school work, play, and may support a communication system. This system may range from "yes/no" words pasted on the tray to an extensive electronic communication device. If the arms of the wheelchair are too high or too low for effective use of the tray, adjustments must be made. When the arms are too high, the padded arm rests of the wheelchair may be removed to lower the tray, or a padded seat may be inserted to raise the child. When the arms are too low, two blocks may be placed under the tray where it contacts the arms of the wheelchair.

The size of the tray depends on its use. A smaller tray is acceptable if used only for supporting books in school, eating, or playing. However, when using an extended communication system, the speech/language pathologist will need a larger surface. A raised edge around the tray will prevent objects from falling and provides space for an eye gaze number system, allowing the flat surface of the tray to be used exclusively for alphabet, vocabulary, and phrases.

The width of the tray must be kept within hand reach or easy eye gaze and should permit passage through doorways. If printing or pictures are used on the board, a cover made of 1/8-inch clear plexiglass will extend the life of the material.

A tray should never extend beyond the outer edge of the footplates because such a tray would change the chair's center of gravity and make it tip easily when pressure is exerted on the edge of the tray.

Large trays have better balance when they extend a couple of inches beyond the back upright of the chair. It is in this area that barrel bolts are placed to insert into the holes that have been drilled in the steel frame on each side of the chair. No space should be allowed between the chair frame and the tray in order to eliminate any sliding movement of the tray.

Upper Body Control

Shoulder, arm, and head control is dependent on the stability maintained in the hips and trunk. The severely involved cerebral palsied child frequently assumes a posture of elbows flexed and hands out to the side at shoulder height. The trunk and head may be extended or dropped forward. For the severely involved child, movement of the head and/or the eyes may be their only functional activity (Figure 8.6). Adaptations added to wheelchairs for control of lower trunk and hips emphasize stability, whereas additions for the upper extremities must strike a balance between stability and function (Guess, 1978).

Monitoring chair adaptations to adjust for growth and function is ongoing. Particular attention must be given the upper extremities because fine skills may start to develop when arms and head are in proper alignment, and seating changes may be required as a result.

Wings. Forward rotation of the shoulders will assist in alignment of the head. Children whose arms are forced out and back by abnormal reflex activity assume an even more abnormal posture when actively trying to move.

The shoulders and arms may be controlled in a forward position when wooden wings are attached to the solid back of the wheelchair. These should extend between the top of the shoulder to the elbow and come forward to the end of the extended upper arm (Figure 8.7). Care should be taken to ensure that the wings hold the upper arms in a forward position without squeezing the shoulders together.

Wings may also be used on either side of the head to keep the head in midline. They should be located to give support without restricting vision. Switches to be operated by head movements may be attached to head wings for controlling communication devices, environmental aids, and toys.

Shoulder Straps. If the head falls forward due to trunk weakness, shoulder straps may be valuable. They are attached to the back of the chair slightly lower than the shoulder and brought forward over the chest to the hip strap. An "H" style (Figure 8.7) is more comfortable than the "V" style, which angles from the shoulders to the hip strap and may cause discomfort in the neck area.

Side Supports. Extensive trunk weakness will require additional side control. Small flat boards may be placed on one or both sides, depending on the trunk position. This surface should be padded and large enough to hold the body in a comfortable, upright alignment.

Figures 8.6 and 8.7 demonstrate the need for special seating and show how easy-to-construct homemade equipment added to the standard wheelchair improves posture and provides stability for children with severe cerebral palsy.

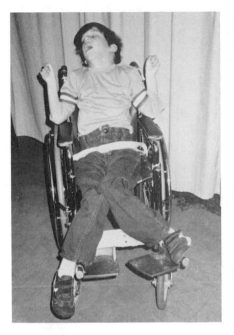

Figure 8.6.
Upright position—unmodified seating.

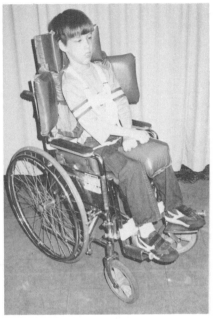

Figure 8.7.
Upright position—modified seating.

Other Types of Seating Equipment

In addition to wheelchairs that have been customized by special inserts, other types of seating should be provided whenever possible (Bergen, 1974). A regular wooden chair, sturdy enough to contain some customized additions, will enable a child to join a group at a table in the classroom or in the dining room. Due to the limited adaptations that can be added to regular chairs, only children who have some trunk and head control will be able to use them successfully.

Roll Seats. This seating arrangement consists of a padded roll with a solid back support (Figure 8.8). When a child straddles the roll, hip abduction is facilitated (Bergen, 1974). Roll seats may be moved anywhere in the classroom when fitted with small casters. If the roll seat is too wide, the legs will internally rotate to an abnormal hip and leg position and could be uncomfortable. Children who assume the frog position should not be considered for a roll seat.

Toilet Seats. A chair-type toilet seat that sits on its own legs over the commode may be fitted with most of the adaptations previously suggested for use with the wheelchair. A safety strap is also highly recommended for toilet seats. A seat of this type is safe and comfortable and provides privacy since the constant attention of an attendant is not required.

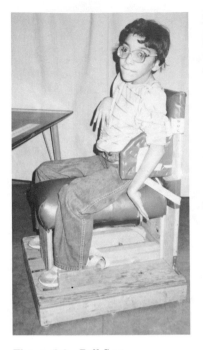

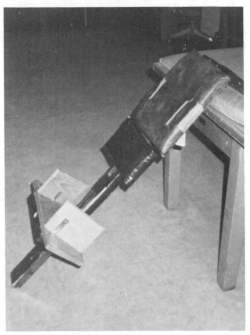

Figure 8.8. Roll Seat.   **Figure 8.9.** Prone stander.

Prone Standers.   For those who can be placed in a weight-bearing position, the prone stander will provide support for correct body alignment. The prone board may be constructed on an "A" frame with its own table tray attached, or it may be leaned on a high table so the child will be able to use that surface for normal activities (Figure 8.9). Adjustable footplates permit it to be used by children of various sizes. A prone board is not indicated for children with poor upper trunk and head control and cannot be used when extreme spasticity or contractures are present. Wide straps for controlling the hips and lower extremities assist in body alignment and stability, thus facilitating some arm use.

AIDS FOR EDUCATION AND COMMUNICATION

As posture improves with proper seating, possibilities for functional movement are seen as arms are freed from total body movement. However, reduced tactile sensation, poor grasp and release, limited range of motion in the forearm, and overflow to the entire body when fine skills are attempted, necessitate the use of adaptive devices.

Holders for Pencils and Papers

It is often difficult for the child with cerebral palsy to hold a paper for drawing or writing. Papers may be taped to a surface or attached to a clipboard with a rubberized surface to prevent sliding. The angle of papers or books can be adjusted by using an easel with the tilt determined by trial and observation.

It is difficult for children with poor arm and hand control to handle pencils and crayons. Thick pencils which are standard items in many classrooms are easier to grasp than regular pencils. They can be made even thicker by wrapping them with sponge and tape. Limited range of motion in the forearm prevents the child from holding a pencil in the standard manner. Adding a hand grip (Figure 8.10) will permit the pencil to contact the paper even when the hand is held with the palm down, or by using a spring clothespin to hold the pencil, the child may grip the "legs" of the clothes pin and control the pencil in this manner.

A molded hand support may be designed by an occupational therapist if more extensive control is needed. Holding a pencil in this manner allows the child to see his or her own handiwork.

When the hands are not capable of being used for writing or even pointing, a headstick may be a possible alternative if the head is sufficiently controllable (Figure 8.11). The cap for the headstick is molded by the occupational therapist, with a medal rod coming from the forehead area (Philpot, 1975). The placement and length of the rod must permit contact with paper using the most relaxed head position possible. The pencil is attached to the rod and may be alternated with the rubber tip for turning pages or pointing to words on a language board. It is also used successfully for typing, operating electronic communication devices, and computers. When head control is insufficient to use a pointing device, an Optical Light Indicator is highly recommended. This device is attached to a band around the head and produces a small beam of light that may be aimed at items on the communication board to indicate word selection.

COMMERCIAL EQUIPMENT

Although most of the equipment and adaptations discussed in this chapter are constructed noncommercially using individual specifications, there are many companies now producing well made equipment with optional items designed for appropriate positioning (Bergen & Colangelo, 1982). No company is able to produce individual customization from stock items for every nuance of posture resulting from a central nervous system disorder, but optional items such as wings, wedges, side supports, seats, and backs may be purchased if carefully selected.

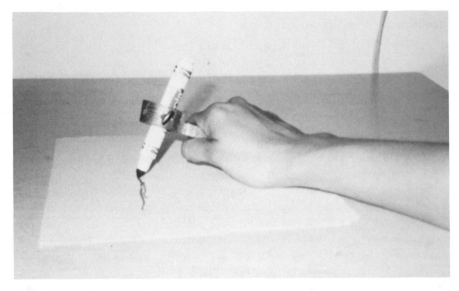

Figure 8.10. Hand grip.

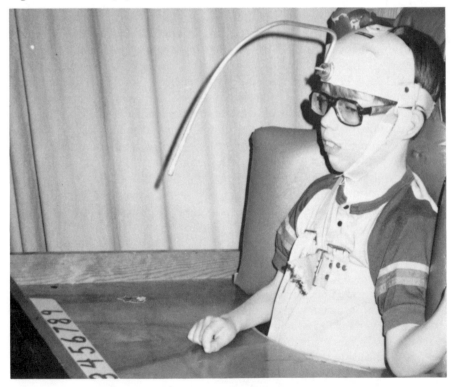

Figure 8.11. Headstick.

After a discriminating selection has been made and the adaptation still does not produce the desired positioning, a combination of commercially produced and clinically designed adaptations could produce the desired alignment.

Commercial items should be approached with caution. Based upon experience, side panels attached to chairs with set screws may not hold after a short period of use, the metal may be too soft to hold the threads for screws, footplates may not accommodate to a 90° angle position, and shoulder straps may not fit properly.

Trays. Many commercial trays are unsatisfactory for purposes other than elbow resting or holding a plate. Extensive communication systems require a much larger surface area, which is difficult to find in commercial trays. A clear acrylic tray may be used to permit sight of lower extremities, thus enhancing body image, but they can be a great distraction to anyone with perceptual difficulty when involuntary movement of the lower extremities is involved.

Chairs. Many types of specialized wheelchairs are available and should be considered. Various chairs that are molded to the individual may be beneficial, but service should be conveniently available for remolding the seating for growth. Roll seats and prone boards, as well as side lyers, are listed in most catalogs providing pediatric equipment. Although expensive, they are useful when carefully selected for size and usage.

Bathroom Needs. Bathing in a tub is made possible by bathing slings. This item will not eliminate the necessary lifting, but will control the body once it is placed in the tub. If the size and weight of the individual are a problem, hydraulic lifts are available.

Commode seats from a catalog are often lacking in the control needed to stabilize a severely handicapped person. An individually designed seat using the principles of good aligned positioning provides more independence, as well as better stability and comfort.

Whenever commercial equipment is being utilized, a close relationship must exist between the vendor and the clinic and/or home in order to create an understanding for the special needs of the individuals involved. This will facilitate proper maintenance and usage.

There will be increased opportunity for persons with cerebral palsy to improve their lifestyle if each person who works or lives with handicapped individuals becomes knowledgeable about the principles of handling, positioning, and the proper use of adaptive equipment.

REFERENCES

Bergen, A. (1974). *Selected equipment for pediatric rehabilitation.* Vahalla, NY: Blythsdale Children's Hospital.

Bergen, A., & Colangelo, C. (1982). *Positioning the client with central nervous system deficits* (Appendix). Vahalla, NY: Vahalla Rehabilitation Publications.

Bobath, D. (1972). *Treatment versus education*. London: Western Cerebral Palsy Centre.

Finnie, N. (1970). *Handling the young cerebral palsied child at home*. New York: E. P. Dutton.

Guess, V. (1978). Central control inefficiency—extraneous motion. *Journal of the American Physical Therapy Association, 58*, 257–404.

Hildreth, K., Horsman, C., & Slurtevante, E. (1982). *Wheelchair training protocol*. Providence, RI: Rhode Island Easter Seal Society.

Hulme, J., Poor, R., Schulein, M., & Pezzino, J. (1983). Perceived behavioral changes observed with adapted seating devices and training programs for multihandicapped, developmentally disabled individuals. *Physical Therapy, 63*, 1429–1433.

Letts, R. (1983). *Goals for seating in cerebral palsy*. Paper presented at the meeting of the International Seating Symposium, New York.

Philpot, R. (1975). Headstick helmet for cerebral palsied children. *American Journal of Occupational Therapy, 29*, 291–292.

CHAPTER 9

Speech Production Problems

Eugene T. McDonald

> *While noting that the act of speaking is influenced by cogni-*
> *tive function and emotional states, McDonald stresses that the*
> *major speech production problems in cerebral palsy arise*
> *from poor neuromuscular control of the speech-producing*
> *mechanism.*

1. *How does speech breathing differ from nonspeech breath-*
   ing, and why do many cerebral palsied children have
   difficulty developing a speech-breathing pattern?
2. *What are the effects of an inadequate speech-breathing*
   pattern on phonation and articulation?
3. *In what ways does poor* laryngeal *control affect the*
   generation of aerodynamic *energy needed for speech*
   production; quasi-periodic acoustic *energy?*
4. *How are resonation and articulation affected by poorly*
   developed antigravity extension?
5. *How does McDonald support his contention that there*
   can be no overall plan for treating speech disorders
   associated with cerebral palsy?
6. *List techniques for improving (a) respiratory control,*
   (b) laryngeal function, and (c) articulation.

INTRODUCTION

It is to be expected that many persons with cerebral palsy would have difficulty producing intelligible speech. By definition, cerebral palsy is a motor disability resulting from brain dysfunction. Speech, to use Kent's (1983) phrase, "is a brisk motor activity" (p. 253). In addition to being "brisk," it is a complex motor activity requiring the coordinated function of more than 50 pairs of muscles. Speech production shares this musculature with several other physiological processes such as respiration, laryngeal valving, chewing, sucking, and swallowing. In the past, speech production was viewed as an "overlaid function" with speech movements developing as refinements of the earlier appearing vegetative movements. Research now suggests that, while speech and vegetative movements are subserved by some common neural structures, speech production is controlled by neurophysiologic mechanisms which are unique to humans and are distinct from the mechanisms involved in vegetative acts (Hixon & Hardy, 1964; Netsell, 1981).

The major speech problem seen in cerebral palsy is *dysarthria*. Early definitions (e.g., Travis, 1971) described dysarthria as an "articulatory disorder due to impairment of the part of the central nervous system which directly controls the muscles of articulation." This definition is now regarded as inadequate. Motor speech problems may result from peripheral nerve lesions as well as CNS lesions. Not only articulation is affected, but other aspects of speech production—respiration, phonation, resonance and prosody—are also impaired. The symptoms of dysarthria vary depending on the site of lesion; hence, the term refers to a group of speech disorders with various symptoms resulting from a lesion in the central or peripheral nervous systems (Darley, Aronson, & Brown, 1975). The symptoms may also vary in severity. Neurologic impairment may be so slight that it is not suspected as the cause of a speech problem. Severe neurologic dysfunction may preclude the possibility of developing intelligible speech. In Chapter 1 cerebral palsy is defined as a condition characterized by motor dysfunction resulting from brain pathology which occurred before, during, or shortly after birth. The dysarthrias of cerebral palsy are manifestations of intracranial pathology. Beyond this gross statement there has been much speculation concerning the neurological bases but, as Neilson and O'Dwyer (1981) point out, "There has been little experimental verification of the existing theories concerning the pathophysiology of dysarthria in cerebral palsy."

Dysarthria is to be distinguished from apraxia of speech which is also a speech production problem caused by a CNS lesion. Like dysarthria the pathophysiology of apraxia is not well understood but it is thought that apraxia is a problem of motor planning. Apraxia of speech will show up primarily in articulation and may be a component of the total speech

production problem in cerebral palsy. When present, apraxia would interfere with voluntary efforts to move or position structures involved in
production of speech sounds.

PRODUCTION OF SPEECH

Speaking cannot be separated from cognitive functions. One speaks about
something. The content of an utterance and how the utterance is formulated linguistically are nonmotor aspects of the speech act. Production
of the sounds of speech is a motor act designed to direct a flow of air into
the vocal tract where consonants and vowels are formed by action of laryngeal, pharyngeal, and oral musculature. The speech producing mechanism
consists of three components—respiratory, laryngeal, and supralaryngeal.

Respiratory Functions

The basic function of the respiratory system is to supply oxygen to the
blood and to remove carbon dioxide. The expiratory phase of respiration
also provides the aerodynamic energy needed for speech production. Respiration is an exceedingly complex process, but a detailed understanding
of respiratory physiology is not necessary for our purpose. We need to know
the simple mechanics of inspiration and expiration and how speech breathing differs from vegetative breathing.

A basic physical law accounts for the flow of air in the respiratory
system: When the volume of a gas is enlarged, its pressure falls and, conversely, when the volume of a gas is decreased, its pressure increases. The
highly elastic lungs are located within the thorax and connected to the
atmosphere via the trachea, larynx, and supralaryngeal cavities. The size
of the thoracic cage can be enlarged or contracted. When enlarged, lung
volume increases, pressure of the air within the lungs drops below
atmospheric pressure and air flows through the nose or mouth into the
lungs. Contraction of the thoracic cage decreases the volume of the lungs
and raises the air pressure, thus causing air to flow from the lungs through
the trachea, larynx, pharynx, and out the nose or mouth. Descent of the
diaphragm in inspiration increases the vertical dimension of the thorax.
Two features of the ribs account for a side-to-side increase: the angle at
which the ribs attach to the spine and the sternum, and the curvature
of the ribs. When raised in inhalation, the curvature increases the distance between corresponding ribs on the right and left side. As the ribs
pivot on the spine, they cause an upward and forward movement of the
sternum, thus increasing the anterior-posterior dimension of the thorax.

Several factors operate to contract the thoracic cage. At the termination of inhalation, the muscles which contracted to elevate the ribs against
gravity relax, and gravity operates to cause the ribs to fall. As the ribs

are elevated in inhalation, the cartilages by which they are attached to the sternum are twisted. Untwisting of the costal cartilages contributes to returning the ribs to their lower position. The elastic tissues of the lungs recoil after being stretched. Descent of the diaphragm displaces the abdominal viscera and stretches the abdominal musculature. With relaxation of the diaphragm at the end of inhalation, the viscera return to their former position aided by contraction of abdominal musculatures. Observations of normal breathing in an infant would reveal a predominance of abdominal activity, partly because the mechanisms for thoracic expansion are not yet developed. The ribs of infants are attached almost perpendicularly to the spine, allowing little possibility for the elevation which produces lateral and anterior-posterior expansion of the thoracic cage. As the child grows, the ribs slant downward from the spine making elevation possible. Observations of normal breathing in an older child would reveal simultaneous increases in abdominal and thoracic circumferences during inhalation and simultaneous decreases during exhalation.

In quiet breathing, inhalation and exhalation are about equal in duration. In contrast to this tidal flow, speech breathing consists of "extremely abrupt inspirations and considerably prolonged expirations." These changes in the breathing cycle are "embodied in differences with regard to timing, volume events, pressure events and musculature control" (Hixon, Mead, & Goldman, 1976). In speech breathing, inspiration requires about one-sixth of the breathing cycle. During the remaining five-sixths of the cycle, controlled exhalation maintains the relatively uniform air pressure level required for production of connected speech. To maintain a uniform level as air flows from the lungs into the vocal tract requires fine adjustments in the force applied by the respiratory musculature (Daniloff, Schuckers, & Feth, 1980).

Nonspeech breathing is controlled by a respiratory center located in the brainstem. In response to the level of carbon dioxide in the blood and the degree to which the lungs are extended, this center reflexively initiates and terminates inhalation. The respiratory mechanism is also responsive to stimulation of other sensory receptors (e.g., cold applied to the skin, inhalation of vapors such as ammonia, irritation of nose or throat, or various sights and sounds). Respiration is subject to cortical control for speech production and singing. Through conscious control it is possible to arrest breathing, and to change respiratory rate or the depth of inspiration; however, we are usually not conscious of respiratory function at rest or during speech production.

Respiratory Problems in Cerebral Palsy.   Only a few studies of speech breathing in cerebral palsy have been published. Hardy (1964) studied the following aspects of respiration in 18 spastic quadriplegics, 15 athetoids, and 33 normal children matched by height: rate of rest breathing, minute ventilation, tidal volume, expiratory reserve, inspiratory reserve, and vital capacity measured in supine, sitting, and prone. He concluded, on the basis of comparison of means, that differences in posture had no effect on respiratory function for spastics, athetoids, or controls, and he found "no evidence from this study that hyperactive righting reflexes are generally present in conditions of spasticity and athetosis, at least in so far as those reflexes are manifested in neuromotor patterns of respirations."

In Chapter 7, Alexander described how abnormal distribution of flexor and/or extensor muscle tone in infants and young children creates skeletal and neuromuscular adjustments which interfere with development of normal respiratory mechanics with detrimental impact on speech development. We have observed several patterns of respiratory mechanics which interfere with speech production in some older cerebral palsied children.

1. *Failure to develop a speech breathing pattern consisting of quick inhalation and prolonged, controlled exhalation.* When these children attempt to speak, they do so on the expiratory portion of the rest breathing cycle. With a rapid rest respiratory rate, expiration may be of too short duration to support speech production, especially if the child has poor laryngeal and oral motor control. Often these children cannot voluntarily hold their breath momentarily or prolong exhalation. It appears that brain stem level respiratory control is present but the cortical control needed for speech production has not developed.

2. *Antagonistic diaphragmatic-abdominal and thoracic movements.* This condition is also referred to as "reversed breathing" or "asynchronous breathing." Normally, the thoracic and abdominal circumferences increase simultaneously in inhalation. While the rib cage rises, the diaphragm descends as they work together to increase the volume of the thorax. Some persons with cerebral palsy do not develop, or are unable to maintain, this coordinated thoracic and diaphragmatic activity. When the diaphragm descends for inhalation, the rib cage descends also, thus limiting the increase of thoracic volume. In exhalation the diaphragm ascends but the rib cage elevates also. It is difficult for these persons to produce the aerodynamic energy required for speaking.

3. *Poor neuromuscular control of prolonged exhalation.* As noted earlier, a relatively uniform level of air pressure during exhalation is required for production of connected speech. At the beginning of an utterance of normal loudness, pressure is created by the elastic contraction of the lungs with no checking or braking effort by the chest wall (rib cage, diaphragm, and abdomen) musculature. As the elastic contraction force decreases, the musculature of the rib cage, diaphragm, and abdomen work "in concert to raise the overall pressure of the chest wall gradually and in systematic

relationship to the decreasing relaxation pressure which accompanies decreasing lung volume" (Hixon et al., 1976). For many cerebral palsied speakers the expiratory musculature does not work "in concert" and the relationship to decreasing relaxation pressure is not systematic. Resulting utterances are characterized by poor prosody, especially inappropriate variations in loudness.

Laryngeal Functions

Air leaving or entering the lungs must pass through the larynx, which sits above the trachea and opens into the pharynx. The larynx has two main functions. First, it operates as a valve to protect the trachea and lungs against entrance of solids or liquids during swallowing. This is achieved by adduction of the vocal folds to produce a cover over the trachea and by elevating the larynx toward the epiglottis which is tipped to deflect food and fluid away from the larynx and toward the esophagus. In Chapter 7, Alexander described how this function is disturbed in children with neuromuscular dysfunction.

A second function is related to the production of speech. If the vocal folds are fully abducted, the exhaled air passes noiselessly through larynx as in the production of voiceless speech sounds. For whispering the vocal folds are brought closer together creating a constriction through which the exhaled air passes, adding a random noise type of acoustic energy to the aerodynamic energy of exhalation. When the adducted folds obstruct the flow of air from the lungs, pressure rises until the folds are blown apart. Pressure is then released and the folds come together again only to be blown apart when the subglottal pressure rises sufficiently. This complex process, known as phonation, is the source of the quasi-periodic acoustic energy characteristic of voiced speech sounds (Daniloff et al., 1980; Heinz, 1974). By approximating the vocal folds more strongly, a greater subglottal pressure is required to force them apart thus increasing the loudness of voice. Pitch of voice is varied by changing vocal fold tension—the more tension in the folds, the higher the pitch.

Laryngeal Problems in Cerebral Palsy. In Chapter 7, Alexander described how neuromotor dysfunction which restricts or prevents the development of active, coordinated antigravity movements directly affects respiration and phonation. She stressed the interrelatedness of respiration, vocal fold, and oral motor activities. In older children and adults, several types of laryngeal dysfunction may be observed.

Failure to Coordinate Phonation With Exhalation. In some individuals the vocal folds are open during exhalation, making phonation impossible. If the folds are abducted during the early part of exhalation, air leaks rapidly leaving little for speaking when adduction is achieved. This is a critical problem when expirations are short or poorly controlled.

Excessively Strong Adduction of Vocal Folds. If the vocal folds are too tightly approximated, the subglottal pressure may not be strong enough to separate them and initiate phonation. The individual may be seen to posture the mouth as if to speak but no sound is produced. In cases where the vocal fold closure is less excessive but still too strong, a higher level of expiratory pressure will move the vocal folds, but vocal loudness will be inappropriate.

Poorly Regulated Vocal Fold Tension. Frequency of vocal fold vibration is determined primarily by vocal fold tension. The greater the tension, the faster the vocal folds vibrate and the higher the pitch of the voice. In normal speaking, tension is varied to produce intonation patterns which carry some of the meaning of an utterance. Questions, for example, are usually spoken with a rising pitch at the end of the utterance, whereas the pitch falls at the end of a declarative statement. Persons who cannot vary vocal fold tension speak in a monotone. Those who cannot control tension changes have inappropriate pitch variations.

Inappropriate Timing of Phonation. Normally the onset and termination of phonation is precisely timed to the production of voiced sounds. In cerebral palsy extraneous phonations, which have no relation to the utterance, sometimes occur. Farmer and Lencione (1977) have called attention to *prevocalization*, (i.e., phonation of a vowel-like sound prior to articulation). Voicing errors on cognates are frequent (Platt, Andrews, & Howie, 1980).

Supralaryngeal Functions

The pharyngeal, oral, and nasal spaces and the structures therein comprise the upper respiratory tract, the upper portion of the alimentary canal, and also the vocal tract. These supralaryngeal structures and spaces are involved in breathing, sucking, chewing, and swallowing and in the production of speech. Two aspects of speech production occur above the level of the larynx—resonation and articulation. These functions are interrelated.

The tone generated at the larynx consists of a fundamental frequency plus a number of overtones. When this sound enters the pharynx, mouth, and sometimes the nose, it is modified since these cavities, acting as resonators, reinforce those frequencies to which they are tuned. Damping of some frequencies may also occur. The soft palate may couple or uncouple the nasal cavity and movements of the lips, tongue, and mandible change the size of oral and oral pharyngeal cavities and their openings. The length and diameter of the pharynx may be varied. These changes affect overall voice quality and differentiations among speech sounds.

The air stream is also modified by the lips, mandible, and tongue as these structures move to constrict or occlude the airflow at various places in the vocal tract, a process called "articulation." Constrictions are sources of acoustic energy of the random noise type, and occlusions are sources of pressure-release acoustic energy. The energy source employed, (i.e., the *manner* of production) determines the *class* of sound produced. Vowels and voiced sounds employ quasi-periodic sources of acoustic energy; sibilants and fricatives employ random noise; plosives employ pressure release. In producing some sounds, two energy sources are used, (e.g., a voiced plosive employs the quasi-periodic and the pressure-release source). The *sound within the class* (which vowel, which plosive, which sibilant) is determined by size and location of the resonating cavities *within the vocal tract* which is determined by *the place* or location of the obstruction to the airstream. A posterior resonating cavity extends from the glottis to the point where the airstream is obstructed, and an anterior cavity extends from that point to the mouth opening.

A brief review of how consonants and vowels are classified will facilitate discussion of supralaryngeal problems in cerebral palsy and treatment techniques. Vowels are usually classified according to whether the high point of the tongue is in the back, middle, or front of the mouth (Figure 9.1). An additional lingual feature is the shape of the tongue— convex or concave. Tongue positioning and shaping for vowels is effected largely by extrinsic lingual musculature and, in comparison to most consonants, the movements are gross (Perkell, 1969). However, a high degree of lingual control is required to produce recognizable differentiations among even the commonly used vowels. The amount of mandibular depression increases as the height of the tongue varies from high to low. In normal speech, this depression is *finely graded* with the jaw dropping only a few millimeters as a speaker produces, progressively from high to low, either the front or back vowel series. Lip movements are also involved in vowel production. For the mid-vowels, the lips merely separate as the mandible depresses. For the front vowels, the angles of the mouth retract to various degrees to produce an elongated orifice from side to side, and for the back vowels the opening movement is accompanied by various degrees of lip protrusion. Again, it is to be noted that there is a finely graded retraction of the lips as the front vowels are produced progressively from low to high and a finely graded protrusion as the back vowels are produced from low to high. Mandibular movement, labial movement, and lingual movement are coordinated in vowel production to create the appropriate configuration of resonating cavities for each vowel.

Consonants may be classified according to three factors: *manner, place,* and *voicing.*

Manner determines the class of sound produced, and refers to the degree to which the articulators impede the outgoing air stream. Complete obstruction stops the airflow allowing pressure to build up which, when released, produces a sound of the *plosive* class. Consonants produced

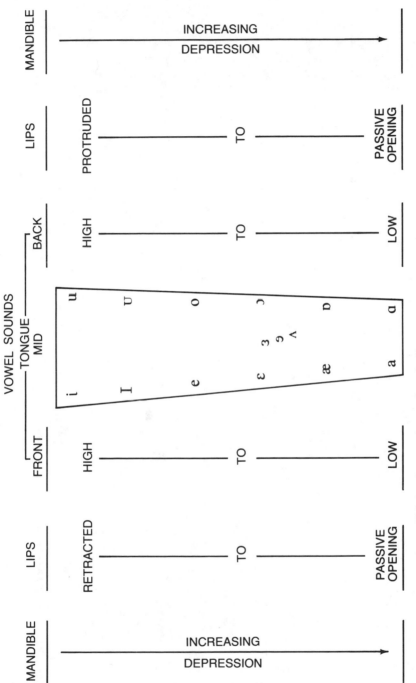

Figure 9.1. Lip, tongue, and mandible involvement in vowel production.

MANNER OF PRODUCING ACOUSTIC ENERGY
(determines class of sound)

		—stop—						—continuant—					
	plosive			fricative			affricative			nasal		glide	
	v	u		v	u		v	u		v		v	u
Bi-labial	b	p								m		w	ʍ
Labio-dental				v	f								
Lingua-dental				ð	θ								
Alveolar	d	t		z	s		dʒ	tʃ		n		l	
				ʒ	ʃ								
Palatal												r	
												j	
Velar	g	k								ŋ			
Glottal					h								

v-phonated or voiced   uv-without phonation or unvoiced

TARGET AREA OF ARTICULATORS
(determines specific sound within class)

Figure 9.2. Class and within-class classification of consonants.

by a continuous flow of air are classified as *continuants*. This class is sub-divided on the basis of the degree to which the airflow is impeded, (i.e., the amount of constriction in the vocal tract). Sibilants are produced when air is forced through a small aperture resulting in a hissing sound. A slightly lesser constriction produces fricatives; affricates are slowly released stop consonants. Vowels and vowel-like sounds are produced when the constriction is not great enough to generate random noise. In producing nasals there is a continuous flow of air through the nasal passages but none through the mouth. A high degree of fine oral motor control is required to produce the several degrees of obstruction ranging from complete closure to relatively complete openness.

Place of articulation determines which sound within a class is produced. In this classification two factors are considered: (a) the location within the vocal tract where the occlusion or constriction occurs, and (b) which articulatory structure impedes the airstream. The place of artic-ulation is a target area rather than a specific spot. When speaking at a conversational rate, undershooting and overshooting of the target area for a phoneme occur, but gross misses result in failure to produce the intended speech sound. Both intrinsic and extrinsic lingual muscles are involved in moving the tongue toward target areas and creating the proper degree of obstruction. Mandibular movements are coordinated with tongue and labial movements to produce consonants but the extent of mandibu-lar depression is less than 15 mm for the average speaker.

Voicing, the presence or absence of phonation, is a laryngeal, rather than a supralaryngeal, process. It is discussed here because it is consid-ered in classifying consonants. Voicing is not graded, (i.e., sounds are either voiced or unvoiced). Since, in connected speech, voiced sounds may be preceded or followed by voiceless sounds, the initiation and termination of phonation must be precisely timed. This not only requires control of the adductors and abductors of the larynx, but close coordination with movements of the supralaryngeal structures as well.

Supralaryngeal Problems in Cerebral Palsy. In Chapter 7, Alex-ander described how abnormal and compensatory head/neck posture and oral-motor functions develop as a result of abnormal muscle tone. These abnormal postures and movements later result in abnormal resonation and articulation.

Resonance Problems. Hyperextension of the head and neck accom-panied by extreme depression of the mandible is frequently seen in cere-bral palsy. These postures alter the size of oral and pharyngeal cavities, resulting in the creation of abnormal resonance characteristics. Mandibu-lar depression pulls the back of the tongue downward and, because of the muscular connections between the tongue and soft palate, this interferes with the palatal movement required to close the nasopharyngeal port. In some cases control of the velopharyngeal musculature is not well developed. Unwanted nasal resonance occurs. Excessive mandibular depression and poor neuromuscular control of the tongue make it difficult to produce the resonating cavities by which vowels are given distinctiveness. Another factor which affects vocal tract cavity size is the attempt to compensate for failure of the velopharyngeal mechanisms to close the opening into the nasal cavity (McDonald & Koepp-Baker, 1951; Netsell, 1969). To generate more oral resonance when the nasal cavity is coupled to the vocal tract, the cerebral palsied speaker increases the size of the oral pharyngeal cavity by depressing the mandible and the tongue. This adjustment changes but does not normalize resonance. It also adversely affects articulation. Resonance problems range from mild, such as slight nasality or vowel distortions, to severe ones which adversely affect production of virtually all sounds. A combination of uncontrolled loudness and inappropriate resonance degrades speech intelligibility and has an unfavorable effect on listeners.

Articulation Problems. The subprocesses of speech production (respiration, phonation, resonation, articulation) are closely interrelated. Because the system functions in a unitary manner, to consider articulation independently may lead to oversimplification and inaccurate assessment of the speech production problem (Hardy, 1983). When observing oral motor functions, one must bear in mind that malfunctions in other parts of the system also contribute to the characteristics of the speech produced.

Mandibular movements and postures are frequently disturbed. A major problem is hyperdepression (also referred to as hyperextension) which may be so extreme as to cause the condyle of the mandible to slip out of the temperomandibular fossa (Palmer, 1948). When the mandible is hyperdepressed, the lips are pulled apart and stretched, making it difficult or impossible to approximate, protrude, or retract as required for production of various speech sounds. Excessive depression of the mandible draws the tongue downward and prevents it from reaching target areas and producing the necessary occlusions and constrictions.

A variety of abnormal lingual movements and postures are seen in children with cerebral palsy. Some allow production of consonants but they are often misarticulated. At the other extreme, impaired lingual movement may allow production of only a few vowel-like sounds because the tongue cannot assume the proper shape nor approach the proper target area for production of a recognizable vowel. Clinically, it appears that there is a direct relationship between the complexity of neuromuscular action required to produce a sound and the likelihood of misarticulation.

Rutherford (1939) and Byrne (1959) studied the articulation of groups of spastic and athetoid children. Examination of their data indicates that

the sounds most frequently misarticulated are the lingua-alveolar fricatives and the lingua-palatal glides. These are the last sounds normally
developing children master and require the greatest complexity of movement for their production (Kent, 1976; Locke, 1972). Occlusive sounds (stop
plosives) are less frequently misarticulated than those requiring constriction. Adult patterns of misarticulation are similar, a finding which led
Platt, Andrews, Young, & Quinn (1980) to conclude, "The apparent stability of these phonetic inadequacies from childhood to adulthood probably
signals the neuromotor limitations which are inherent in the speech
production of persons suffering from cerebral palsy" (p. 38). Phonemic ana-
lyses of the articulation errors of cerebral palsied adults indicate that
within-manner errors occur significantly more frequently than between-
manner errors (Platt, Andrews, & Howie, 1980). For example, the speaker
might produce a plosive but use the incorrect place of articulation for the
intended plosive, or constrict the airway but in the wrong area for the
intended fricative or affricate. In general the tendency of persons who use
defective articulation for communication is to employ movements which
are easy to make in place of those which are more difficult to produce.

Combining Sounds

It is to be emphasized that speech sounds are not independent units
produced by static postures of the articulators. Each sound is coarticulated
with other sounds and, in connected speech, the coarticulated sounds are
grouped in several ways. The most obvious way is to produce words which
convey the meaning of an utterance; however, a word is composed of one
or more syllables which appear to be the production and perceptual units
of speech. The arrangement of sounds within the syllable determines the
syllable shape. The most common shapes are V, CV, VC and CVC. A grouping of syllables which corresponds to a unit of meter in verse is the *foot*.
A foot may contain one or more syllables, only one of which may be stressed.
Another grouping is the *phrase*. In connected speech we often pause, then
begin speaking again on the same exhalation. Pauses are the boundaries
of phrases. A larger grouping is the breath group, the boundaries of which
are the initiation and termination of an exhalation (McDonald, 1980a).

As noted, a *foot* is characterized by differences in syllable stress.
Stressed syllables are of longer duration and increased loudness. These
factors—duration and loudness—along with pitch variations produce the
prosodic characteristics of speech. They are sometimes referred to as
suprasegmental features because they are added to the sound segments.
Problems of Combining Sounds in Cerebral Palsy. Difficulty
ranges from minor prosodic deviations to total inability to produce a
consonant-vowel combination. Production of post-vocalic consonants as
in VC or CVC syllables is difficult for many children who have poor oral

motor control. Utterances are often limited to one or two syllables on an exhalation, thus eliminating the coarticulatory movements which occur across syllable boundaries.

Even in speakers who can utter several syllables in a breath group, prosody might be deviant. Poor control of laryngeal musculature causes pitch variations which result in abnormal intonation patterns. Loudness is determined by tension of the vocal folds and aerodynamic force. When these are poorly controlled, loudness may be inappropriate. To produce the durational differences associated with the perception of stressed and unstressed syllables requires fine grading of articulatory movements. For stressed sounds, articulatory movements are more precise in reaching the appropriate place of articulation. Such control requires stronger neural signals to the speech musculature (Minifie, Hixon, & Williams, 1973) and is beyond the capability of many persons with cerebral palsy. When they attempt to combine sounds in polysyllabic utterances, their intelligibility is poorer than when they produce monosyllables or bisyllables.

FACTORS CONTRIBUTING TO SPEECH PRODUCTION PROBLEMS

The primary cause of poor neuromuscular control of respiratory, laryngeal and supralaryngeal structures is the brain dysfunction which causes faulty motor commands to be sent to the musculature. Closely related are the maladaptive postures of oral structures which develop as the organism attempts to compensate for dysfunction in other parts of the system. Unregulated emotional reactions adversely affect speech production. Slight changes in a social situation can create stress which is often reflected in rising pitch and deteriorating articulation. Some undesirable speech behaviors become habituated and appear even when physical or psychological stress is not present. Low cognitive function is a frequent contributor to delayed and impaired speech development and influences response, rate of progress, and amount gained in therapeutic programs (Parette & Hourcade, 1984). It is common for several of these factors to co-exist, and the influence of each must be considered when developing a treatment program.

REMEDIATION OF SPEECH PROBLEMS

There can be no overall plan for treating the speech disorders associated with cerebral palsy because cerebral palsy is not a homogeneous condition. The combination of contributing factors and the speech symptoms vary from individual to individual. The small groups which have been studied cannot be considered as representative samples of the cerebral palsied population, and conclusions drawn from them cannot be generalized to all persons with cerebral palsy. Therapy outcomes have not been studied, but clinical experience shows the results of therapy range from attaining essentially normal speech to failure to achieve intelligible speech despite many years of intensive speech therapy. In between are many who can make themselves understood but with difficulty. Often prosody remains a problem even for those who learn to articulate the vowels and consonants. Some individuals who have made little progress during childhood learn how to produce understandable speech during adolescence and young adulthood. During treatment, long plateaus in speech improvement followed by brief periods of progress are not uncommon. Speech pathologists often observe these phenomena, but they have not yet been studied. Longitudinal studies are needed to develop prognostic criteria and aid in developing treatment programs.

General Considerations

1. Assessment of the problem is essential before initiating treatment of any type of speech disorder, but this is especially true in cerebral palsy because of the many contributing factors which interfere with speech production and progress in therapy. Information is needed regarding: (a) how, with whom, and about what the child attempts to communicate, (b) level of cognitive function, (c) language development, (d) vision and audition, (e) general neuro-motor development, (f) respiratory, laryngeal, and supra-laryngeal functions especially as related to speech production, (g) psycho-social development, and (h) sources of and reactions to stress. Usually extended observation is necessary to obtain a valid assessment, and techniques such as diagnostic teaching must be used in addition to formal testing.

2. During therapy the child should be positioned to achieve as near normal distribution of muscle tone as possible. For some children speech therapy may begin on a mat or side lyer. Seated children should be supported so their efforts to maintain sitting balance do not interfere with speech breathing, phonation, or development of oral motor control. The speech clinician should sit on a low seat or on the floor so the child can look at his or her face without hyperextending the head and neck.

3. Therapists must be alert to how their behavior influences the child since many children with cerebral palsy overreact to emotionally colored stimuli. A loud voice or laugh, even when meant to convey approval, can disturb the child and interfere with therapy. Overstimulation of the limbic system raises emotional tone and interferes with neuro-muscular control (see Chapter 2).

4. Therapy must be interactive (i.e., what the clinician does next must be related to what the child has just done). The therapist must be alert to and counteract undesirable increases in muscle tone, stress reactions, fatigue, and loss of attention. Short-term goals developed through task analysis enable the therapist to detect and respond to slight changes in the child's performance.

Respiration

Treatment of speech breathing problems begins with the handling and positioning described in Chapters 7 and 8. These procedures attempt to counteract the abnormal muscle tone which affects posture and movement and interferes with respiration and phonation. The following procedures are useful in helping children learn to shift from the nearly equal durations of inhalation and exhalation of rest breathing to the quicker inhalations and controlled exhalations required for speech production.

1. With the child in supine, flexed at knees and hips, elbows flexed with lower arms across the chest, and head and neck flexed, stimulate longer vocalizations. Use light tickling and visual and auditory stimuli to provoke laughter. Encourage the child to imitate your vocalization of a prolonged vowel and a chain of three or four CV syllables such as /ba, ba, ba/ and /ma, ma, ma/.

2. For children who cannot voluntarily inhale more deeply and prolong exhalation, exercises designed to develop cortical control of respiration are indicated. While the child is positioned to normalize tone (e.g., in the supine, flexed position, described above) induce deep inhalation by touching the skin with an ice cube or by momentarily covering the nose and mouth with a tissue. When the therapist has established rapport and has explained what will take place most children accept these procedures without apprehension. The cold stimulus and the brief obstruction of inhalation are followed by several cycles of deeper breathing. Direct the child's attention to the sensations associated with deeper breathing, especially movement of chest and abdominal area. Model a sigh or whispered vowel timed with child's exhalation and encourage imitation. When the child can do this on each of the longer exhalations change the sigh to a phonated low back vowel. Next teach the child to hold the inhaled air until told to exhale slowly. Direct the child's attention to the sensations associated with holding the breath before beginning exhalation. This will increase cortical control. Model and have the child imitate vocalizing a low back vowel on the exhalation. Care must be exercised to avoid creation of unwanted tension by encouraging prolonged vocalizations which require a volume of air not readily available to the child.

After the child acquires control of exhalation, work to develop voluntary control of inhalation. With the child appropriately positioned to normalize tone, raising the arms from the side to above the head aids in expansion of the chest, thus helping the child inhale. Practice in voluntary inhalation, brief holding of breath, followed by controlled exhalation with vocalization will help some children develop a speech breathing pattern. Since these procedures require cognitive development adequate to understand directions and perform the tasks described, they may not be effective with low functioning children.

3. Speakers who have developed a speech breathing pattern but have poor control of exhalation can often improve voice quality and speech intelligibility by limiting the number of syllables produced on an exhalation. As air flows from the lungs during speech, the muscles of exhalation must apply increasing and well-regulated force to push air through the vocal tract at a relatively uniform pressure. Some cerebral palsied speakers can regulate this force only during the early portion of controlled exhalation. As speaking continues, they lose control of the muscles of exhalation with consequent deterioration of speech. By observation determine how many syllables can be uttered before signs of loss of control appear. Increased tension associated with the increased strength of muscle contraction required to generate the aerodynamic energy results in pitch and loudness changes. As the heightened muscle tone spreads throughout the vocal tract, articulation becomes less precise. Through training and practice many cerebral palsied speakers can learn to replenish the air supply by inhaling before hypertonicity develops. This is sometimes referred to as *phrasing*; however, phrases are marked by pauses in the utterance and do not require an inhalation. Since the goal is to maintain an easily controlled volume of air by shortening the exhalation portion of the speech breathing cycle, the focus should be on the *breath group* rather than the *phrase*.

Phonation

Laryngeal and respiratory activities are closely interrelated, hence treatment of problems of phonation is often coordinated with treatment of speech breathing problems.

1. Excessive adductor tone closes the vocal folds tightly, thus interfering with initiation of exhalation and phonation. In children with strong extensor tone the supine flexed position, as described in the discussion of treating speech breathing problems, helps normalize tone. With the child in this position, the therapist can sometimes facilitate phonation by slowly turning the head from side to side as in shaking the head for "no" or forward and backward as in nodding "yes." Attempts to sing simple songs along with the therapist help some children reduce laryngeal tension. Modeling whispered and soft vocalizations for the child to imitate helps some children produce more normal adduction. It is essential to have good

rapport with the child because fear, insecurity, anger, and other feelings contribute to laryngeal tension. Generally speaking, training of this type should continue until the child can easily initiate and sustain phonation.

2. For cerebral palsied speakers who have poor control of pitch and loudness, the use of smaller breath groups is helpful. Through training, many can become aware of their rising pitch and, instead of continuing, pause, inhale, and begin speaking in a more relaxed manner. Emotion and stress frequently result in production of voice which is too high in pitch and too loud. Awareness of this relationship is the first step in the speaker's development of conscious control of pitch and intensity. Some cerebral palsied speakers develop automatic control of pitch and intensity but many must be continually conscious of the nature of their vocal output.

Articulation

It is to be remembered that the supralaryngeal function of articulation produces sounds which are superimposed on an airstream generated by exhalation and modulated by phonation. It is ineffective to focus primarily on articulatory movements when exhalation and phonation are poorly controlled. Also it is to be remembered that positioning of oral structures such as hyperdepression of the mandible and retraction of the tongue may be compensations for poorly developed antigravity extension. General improvement in postural tone may be necessary before adequate articulatory movements can be developed.

1. With cerebral palsied persons whose speech is very difficult to understand because only a few speech sounds are used, training for precise articulation of consonants is usually not effective. However, establishing the correct syllable shape (CV, VC, CVC) improves intelligibility of a word even when the consonant is not articulated correctly (Faircloth & Faircloth, 1970). Intelligibility is further enhanced by producing the correct class of consonant even though it is not the right sound within the class. This means that when the speaker does not use the proper *place* of articulation, effort should be made to use the appropriate *manner* of production. Following is an outline of a treatment program for this type of speech problem:

   a. Record the vowels and consonants which can be identified in a wide sampling of utterances by encircling the appropriate symbol on copies of the vowel and consonant charts shown in Figures 9.1 and 9.2.
   b. If available, use the vowels and consonants in the speaker's production repertoire to develop the correct *syllable shape* for the intended words.
   c. If they are not present, work to establish identifiable productions of two front and two back vowels. Try to avoid excessive mandibu-

lar depression during vowel production by appropriate seating and slight flexion of the head and neck. Combining the vowel with a bilabial consonant in a short series of CV syllables produced as a breath group /ba, ba, ba/ or /ma, ma, ma/ helps limit mandibular depression because the mandible must be elevated for production of the consonant. Practice the CV series with the selected front and back vowels.

    d. Establish at least one consonant of each class and practice with each vowel in CV, VCV, and CVC syllables.

    e. Make a list of the words the speaker attempts. For words which contain sounds the speaker cannot produce, teach a pronunciation substituting sounds of the same class and maintain the correct syllable shape.

2. Even though they have learned to produce all speech sounds, many cerebral palsied speakers have difficulty maintaining good articulation in connected speech. Articulation may be good at the beginning of an utterance but deteriorates as the utterance progresses. A too-rapid rate also adversely affects articulation. By learning to use shorter breath groups and to speak at a slower rate, articulation will be more easily controlled and intelligibility improved.

Until recently, speech/language pathologists emphasized speech training and were reluctant to recommend that communicatively handicapped cerebral palsied persons use communication aids (McDonald, 1980b). We must be careful that today's emphasis on both high and low tech communication aids does not lead to neglect of speech training. While an aid might be the major means of communication for a cerebral palsied person, it is important that the individual be able to produce as many intelligible words as possible. At those times when the aid is not available, the nonspeaking person is frustrated and often isolated. Even for those who cannot achieve precise pronunciations, we should try to develop recognizable approximations of words with high social utility and, when necessary, teach parents, teachers, and associates to recognize these approximations.

REFERENCES

Byrne, M. C. (1959). Speech and language development of athetoid and spastic children. *Journal of Speech and Hearing Disorders, 24,* 231–240.

Daniloff, R., Schuckers, G., & Feth, L. (1980). *The physiology of speech and hearing.* Englewood Cliffs, NJ: Prentice-Hall.

Darley, F., Aronson, A., & Brown, J. (1975). *Motor speech disorders.* Philadelphia: W. B. Saunders.

Faircloth, M. A., & Faircloth, S. R. (1970). An analysis of the articulatory behavior of a speech-defective child in connected speech and isolated-word responses. *Journal of Speech and Hearing Disorders, 35,* 51–62.

Farmer, A., & Lencione, R. (1977). An extraneous vocal behavior in cerebral palsied speakers. *British Journal of Disorders of Communication, 12*, 109–118.

Hardy, J. C. (1964). Lung function of athetoid and spastic quadriplegic children. *Developmental Medicine and Child Neurology, 6*, 378–388.

Hardy, J. C. (1983). *Cerebral palsy*. Englewood Cliffs, NJ: Prentice-Hall.

Heinz, J. M. (1974). Speech acoustics. In T. A. Sebeok (Ed.), *Current trends in linguistics* (Vol. 12) (pp. 2241–2281).

Hixon, T. J., & Hardy, J. (1964). Restricted mobility of the speech articulators in cerebral palsy. *Journal of Speech and Hearing Disorders, 29*, 293–306.

Hixon, T. J., Mead, J., & Goldman, M. D. (1976). Dynamics of the chest wall during speech; function of the thorax, rib cage, diaphragm, and abdomen. *Journal of Speech and Hearing Research, 19*, 297–356.

Kent, R. D. (1976). Anatomical and neuromuscular maturation of the speech mechanism: Evidence from acoustic studies. *Journal of Speech and Hearing Disorders, 19*, 421–447.

Kent, R. D. (1983). Facts about stuttering: Neurophysiologic perspectives. *Journal of Speech and Hearing Research, 48*, 249–255.

Locke, J. L. (1972). Ease of articulation. *Journal of Speech and Hearing Research, 15*, 194–200.

McDonald, E. T. (1980a). Disorders of articulation. In R. J. van Hattum (Ed.), *Communication disorders: An introduction* (pp. 159–206). New York: Macmillan.

McDonald, E. T. (1980b). Early identification and treatment of children at risk for speech development. In R. L. Schiefelbusch (Ed.), Nonspeech language and communication (pp. 49–81). Austin, TX: PRO-ED.

McDonald, E. T., & Koepp-Baker, H. (1951). Cleft palate speech: An integration of research and clinical observations. *Journal of Speech and Hearing Disorders, 16*, 9–20.

Minifie, F. D., Hixon, T. J., & Williams, F. (Eds.).(1973). *Normal aspects of speech and language*. Englewood Cliffs, NJ: Prentice-Hall.

Neilson, P. D., & O'Dwyer, N. J. (1981). Pathology of dysarthria in cerebral palsy. *Journal of Neurology, Neurosurgery, and Psychiatry, 44*, 1013–1019.

Netsell, R. (1969). Changes in oropharyngeal cavity size of dysarthritic children. *Journal of Speech and Hearing Research, 12*, 646–649.

Netsell, R. (1981). The acquisition of speech motor control: A perspective with directions for research. In R. Stark (Ed.), *Language behaviors in infancy and early childhood* (pp. 127–156). New York: Elsevier North Holland.

Palmer, M. (1948). Studies in clinical techniques: Part III. Mandibular facet slip in cerebral palsy. *Journal of Speech and Hearing Disorders, 13*, 44–49.

Parette, H. P., & Hourcade, J. J. (1984). How effective are physiotherapeutic programmes with young mentally retarded children who have cerebral palsy. *Journal of Mental Deficiency Research, 28*, 167–175.

Perkell, J. S. (1969). *Physiology of speech production: Results and implications of a quantitative cineradiographic study*. Cambridge, MA: The MIT Press.

Platt, L. J., Andrews, G., & Howie, P. M. (1980). Dysarthria of adult cerebral palsy; II. Phonemic analysis of articulation errors. *Journal of Speech and Hearing Research, 23*, 41–55.

Platt, L. J., Andrews, G., Young, M., & Quinn, P. (1980). Dysarthria of adult cerebral palsy; I. Intelligibility and articulatory improvement. *Journal of Speech and Hearing Research, 23*, 28–40.

Rutherford, B. R. (1939). Frequency of articulation substitutions in children handicapped by cerebral palsy. *Journal of Speech Disorders, 4*, 285–287.

Travis, L. E. (Ed.). (1971). *Handbook of speech pathology and audiology*. New York: Appleton-Century-Crofts.

CHAPTER 10

Communication Strategies for Infants

Faith Carlson

Carlson writes that the motor dysfunction *and the* cognitive *and* perceptual *problems associated with cerebral palsy can adversely affect development of speech, language, and general communication. Appropriate early intervention is needed to help the infant develop a foundation for the use of symbolic forms of communication.*

1. *Describe how early speech, language, and communication development are affected by motor, cognitive, and perceptual difficulties.*

2. *What arguments does Carlson present for early intervention with children at risk for communication development?*

3. *Several procedures which might be used in evaluating an infant with cerebral palsy are described by Carlson. For each procedure discuss (a) the kind of information it yields, and (b) cautions in using the procedure.*

4. *What does Carlson mean by "parallel communication strategies," and what are the implications of this concept for developing intervention strategies?*

5. *How can (a) the environment, (b) materials, and (c) procedures be modified or adapted to facilitate communication development in the infant with cerebral palsy?*

GENERAL CONSIDERATIONS

Not all children with cerebral palsy experience difficulty in communication development. This chapter will deal more specifically with infants who do encounter problems or appear to be at risk for communication disorders. With infants, it is often difficult to differentiate between a communication disorder and a delayed schedule of development because infancy is marked by rapid changes which vary from child to child. Infant communication assessment instruments are not yet capable of predicting precisely later communication levels. However, speech-language pathologists often can identify those infants who are at risk for normal speech and language development. Some of the identification processes are discussed in this chapter and in Chapter 7.

Decision making regarding the need for early communication intervention is further complicated because it is difficult to make a definite diagnosis of any type in children with suspected neuromuscular dysfunction. Diagnosticians who see infants with possible cerebral palsy may refer a child immediately for communication assessment or may delay for a variety of reasons. They may delay until speech and language have obviously failed to develop normally in order not to concern parents about a problem which may not materialize. In some cases, diagnosticians may fail to address the possibility of a communication problem because they are unaware that intervention can begin in infancy or they have not identified appropriate, available services.

Traditionally, the speech-language pathologists who evaluated and intervened with infants who had cerebral palsy worked on speech development techniques only, or tended to take a "wait-and-see" posture before seeing the children at all. With the advent of more sophisticated augmentative communication strategies, it became possible to adapt these techniques for infants. The speech-language pathologist can now use speech development techniques, augmentative communication strategies, or a combination of both. There is evidence to suggest that nonspeech techniques enhance the chances for speech development rather than interfere with the speech process. Information compiled by Silverman (1980) indicated that in most cases where augmentative communication strategies were used with nonspeaking children and adults, speech attempts either remained the same or increased. Carlson (1981) found that an infant using a combined speech and augmentative communication approach dropped the nonspeech strategies on its own as soon as speech became functional. In light of such information, it may not be wise to use a decision making matrix, such as the one developed by Shane and Bashir (1980) with infants. This matrix suggests using traditional speech techniques before considering augmentative strategies. A combined speech-augmentative communication approach for infants at risk for speech development provides a communication system for the child throughout the developing years without jeopardizing the potential for speech.

Barriers to Communication

The barriers to communication development are as variable as the infants in whom cerebral palsy is manifested and have been covered in detail earlier in this book. Both the motor problems of cerebral palsy and the frequently associated cognitive and perceptual problems can potentially interfere with the child's speech and language development. It is therefore important to identify as early as possible all disorders that are potential barriers to communication. Unfortunately, many of these problems occur in combination, having a compounding rather than an additive detrimental effect on speech and language development.

Motor Problems.   The aberrant movements of cerebral palsy can prevent or distort infants' exploration of their own motion and interfere with environmental interaction. These movements constitute early infant communications, which serve as the basis for later speech and language development (Piaget, 1952; Piaget & Inhelder, 1969). Depending on the physiological site and degree of involvement, their impact on the child's communication will vary.

The Effect on Speech.   Speech requires intricate coordination of muscles which control the movements of breathing, phonation, and articulation. Infants with cerebral palsy may have difficulty performing individual movements or in coordinating movements of the various structures. The manifestations of these problems vary from infant to infant and over time in individual children. Some children experience early and continued feeding or respiratory problems (see Chapters 7 and 9). In other infants, motor problems manifest themselves more subtly, limiting the variety, quality, or quantity of early phonation patterns. The resulting vocal patterns vary from little or no vocalizations other than crying to limited variety in sound patterns, and phonations that are dependent on body position or state.

The Effect on Language.   Language development appears to be affected by the motor problems of cerebral palsy in two distinct ways. First, the infant does not gain the consistent motor experiences that help children discover the underlying concepts later used in language. Second, the infant does not have the quantity of successful soundmaking communication episodes through which children discover the function of language. Many children with motor problems do not have the opportunity to observe environmental changes caused by their own soundmaking or early speech attempts. Infants with cerebral palsy whose journey through the environment is more erratic miss some of these early experiences upon which the semantic and syntactic aspects of language are built. Other infants with cerebral palsy do not miss out on these experiences, but the schedule of their participation is delayed and not in synchrony with their cognitive readiness.

The Effect on General Communication. The motor problems of cerebral palsy can also affect the infant's facial expression, visual tracking, and fixation, as well as the movements read by others as body language. Social communications can be adversely affected from the beginning. Children whose attempts to communicate go unrecognized may never discover that they can initiate control over people and the environment. One infant with a severe asymmetric tonic neck reflex frequently went hungry because the mother misread the child's reflexive turning away as rejection rather than desire for a drink.

Gesturing, gazing, pointing, reaching, and other movements less refined than speech may later be used for augmentative communication. In some infants, the movements needed for these responses may also be distorted, delayed, absent, or bound to specific cues. Only individuals familiar with the child may be able to read those responses.

Perceptual Problems.   Infants with cerebral palsy often display perceptual problems (see Chapters 5 and 6). These perceptual problems may be a result of neuromuscular dysfunction or exist independent of the motor problems. Visual and auditory acuity deficits as well as tactile motokinesthetic feedback problems limit and distort the information received by the child. This further reduces the experiences upon which language can be based. The ability to change focus and shift gaze depends on an intact oculomotor system. The oral-motor dysfunction which results in feeding difficulty and choking can affect eustachian tube functioning and precipitate middle ear problems. These visual and auditory problems may change from time to time and leave the child with variable information upon which to build a communication system.

Cognitive Problems.   The cognitive delays and disorders frequently found in infants with cerebral palsy may be masked by motor or perceptual problems because infants interact with the world in a sensorimotor manner. On the other hand, bright children with cerebral palsy have been misdiagnosed as having cognitive delays because their motor problems were not accommodated during testing.

Circumventing the Barriers

Although it is often not possible to create normal communication experiences for the child with cerebral palsy, many parallel experiences can be provided. Parallel experiences are those with the same intent which are carried out through another mode. For example, the infant unable to initiate a communication act vocally may be able to do so visually if the adults learn to position themselves so they can view, interpret, and respond to gaze communications. The initial vocalizations or gazes may be random on the child's part. With repeated interpretations and appropriate reaction, they become systems upon which symbols for communicating can be built.

Other barriers can be surmounted by adapting the environment so the infants can interact in spite of their problems. The way in which the adult holds the child and special positioning equipment may make the child available for experience (see Chapter 8). Adapting toys and other materials make play experiences available which serve as the basis for language concepts and interactional opportunities.

A Case for Early Intervention

Intervening as soon as problems are diagnosed or when children are identified as being at risk for speech development provides children with a background for language, speech, or augmentative communication. If a "wait-and-see" attitude is taken, months and years of valuable learning time may be lost both by the child and the parents. By starting early, parents can learn skills by the time their child needs to use them. For example, the child in need of signing as a form of communication will need parents who can sign at a higher level than the infant. With early intervention, the parents can learn signing before, rather than with, the child. This will provide a communication environment parallel to that of the speaking child.

In this author's experience, most parents want to know the full extent of their children's disorder as soon as problems are suspected. They find it frustrating to learn first, that the child may not walk, then months or even years later that the child may not talk. Early intervention not only lets the parents know what problems the children are at risk for, but provides them something to do about it.

EVALUATING THE INFANT WITH CEREBRAL PALSY

Evaluating infants with cerebral palsy poses special problems because testing requires that infants exhibit behaviors that can be interpreted as communications. The intent of the atypical behaviors exhibited by infants with cerebral palsy may be the same as those the tests are attempting to tap; however, the communications may go unrecognized. On standardized tests it is often not possible to give the child credit for these equivalent behaviors. Adaptive testing, skilled observation, and parent interviews can supplement the information from standardized tests.

An evaluation may be carried out simply to see if the infant has a communication problem or appears to be at risk for one. Further assessments are needed when a problem exists. These evaluations should outline the extent of the problem and provide a basis for further intervention.

Norm Referenced Tests

Failure on norm referenced tests often qualifies children for special services. However, because of rigid standards for administration, these tests may not be a true assessment of the child's overall communication skills. These tests rely heavily on motor abilities which many infants with cerebral palsy do not have. Receptive as well as expressive communication responses are often equally affected. On the *SICD* (Hedrick, Prather, & Tobin, 1975), for example, children locked into one-side reflex patterns may be aware of sound originating on either side, but be unable to demonstrate localization, an 8-month level skill.

Progress in augmentative communication strategies may not be reflected on reevaluation using norm referenced tests. These tests often serve only as a continuing measure of the impact cerebral palsy has on the child rather than charting progress.

Criterion Referenced Tests

Criterion referenced tests offer more flexibility. Equivalent items relevant to the child's skills and experiences may be substituted rather than restricting assessment to specific materials and procedures. One child who demonstrated the ability to understand and follow one-step commands failed to comply on one norm referenced test because she was not familiar with the materials. She had been tube fed and hospitalized much of her life and was unfamiliar with spoons, miniature toys, and other items used in the norm referenced test. On criterion referenced tests it is often possible to substitute familiar items or alternate procedures that do not violate the intent of specific test items. A more realistic picture of the communication abilities of the child with cerebral palsy may emerge.

Parent Interview Checklists

Parent interviews may be components of a specific test as in the case of the *SICD* (Hedrick et al., 1975) or independent assessment measures like the *REEL* (Bzoch & League, 1971). They may be norm or criterion referenced. Since infant communication is often idiosyncratic and dependent on familiar contextual cues, the parents may be the only ones who will have observed or recognize specific communications. Interview measures are therefore valuable means for gathering communication information.

Parent interview measures may lead to many inaccuracies, however. Parents may have a different interpretation of the questions than do the evaluators, the stress of the evaluative situation may affect recall, and the infant's behaviors may not have been interpreted as communications.

This author found that if potential communication behaviors were described to the parents they often observed them later at home. Ylvisaker (1981) developed an interview measure which utilized a similar but formalized approach which permitted parents to observe the child and complete the form over time at home.

Adaptive Testing for Abilities Versus Disabilities

In adaptive testing, the intent of individual test items or the measure as a whole remains intact; but the materials, response mode, or testing procedures are altered to accommodate the child's perceptual or motor problems. The intent listed for one item on the *SICD* (Hedrick et al., 1975), for example, is "imitation of motor acts." One of the activities is "claps hands." For children with cerebral palsy who cannot bring their hands to midline, this movement is not possible. On adaptive testing, a movement the child can make such as tapping the knee could be substituted. If the intent of the test was to determine if hand clapping is in the child's repertoire of gestures, then no substitution could be made with adaptive test measures.

In adapting test items for infants, caution should be exercised to avoid substituting procedures that are above the child's cognitive level. Wasson, Tynan, and Gardiner (1982) list many excellent adaptive testing methods, one of which is substituting a scanning device when the child does not have a pointing response. Although scanning may be motorically possible for the 8-month-old infant, it would be above the child's level of cognitive functioning and therefore an inappropriate substitute.

The procedures of adaptive testing should be described in the evaluation report so they can be replicated if necessary. Comparison of results obtained through normal and adaptive testing may serve as useful documentation of skills and deficits or provide a basis for intervention techniques.

Discovering the Child's Existing Communication Skills. Observation and informal assessment may be the best means for discovering which behaviors can be viewed as the infant's existing or potential communication *skills*. Through an informal assessment, the evaluator can look for the child's patterns of movement, gaze, and idiosyncratic vocalizations and how the child uses these patterns in relationship to objects, people, and routines.

It is useful to have a format for organizing informal assessment results. George (1983) developed one for infants based on Piaget's sensorimotor Stages I through VI (Piaget, 1952; Piaget & Inhelder, 1969). This author has found that format to be useful in compiling assessment information.

Auditory-Vocal Communication. Assessment of function and coordination of oral-motor integrity, breath regulation, and phonation capabilities is essential. Even disordered auditory-vocal behaviors can serve as a means to communicate. Some children with deviant oral-motor patterns eventually learn to speak intelligibly, although their deviant patterns do not change dramatically. For example, one 18-month-old boy later developed functional speech and acoustically acceptable production of /t/, /d/, /n/, and /l/ although independent tongue elevation did not emerge.

Visual-Motor Communication. Information about the type, size, and placement of visual materials noticed and recognized by infants is essential in assessing visual-motor communication. Furthermore, it is necessary to determine what cues or additional communications are required by the infant to make visual presentations meaningful. For example, infants may recognize their shoes during the dressing process at home or in occupational therapy, but not outside of those contexts.

Motorkinesthetic Communication. The handling and touch of others serve as communication to the young child and, in return, the children's movements communicate to those around them. During the evaluation, movements with gestural potential need to be evaluated in a manner similar to the assessment of oral motor skills in relation to articulatory movements. Again, input from parents and other disciplines such as physical and occupational therapy will be needed.

The manner in which the infant motorically interacts with materials is an important part of the assessment. Movement in combination with objects serves as a foundation for electronic device activation and activities that lead to the development of semantics. For example, normal children at sensorimotor Stage V (12–18 months) put telephone receivers to their ears and push the phone buttons. Through this play activity, a child can develop understanding of what a telephone is and carry out interactions similar to those used when activating many communication devices. By assessing the type of play in which children can participate, valuable communication information can be obtained.

Other Communication. Although other information cues such as taste and smell may communicate, they do not become formal communication systems. Nonetheless, their value as communication cues may be vital for some infants with cerebral palsy. One child, for example, only had a signal for "eat" at home when surrounded by the smells and sounds of the kitchen.

Evaluating the Environment. Information about appropriate positioning and handling of the infant, the objects the child can manipulate, and the skills of the people who interact with the child can be gathered from parents and other staff members. The speech-language pathologist needs to know how well the parents read the child's existing communications, what the parents know about the child's problems and resulting implications, as well as determine any specialized parenting skills before it will be possible to develop an appropriate parent training program. Those skills will vary with each child's needs.

Sampling Reactions to Adaptive Communications. The best way to evaluate the workability of an adaptive communication system, whether that be a symbol system, a procedure for communicating, or a communication device, is to try the system with the child. If the child appears to be ready for symbols, a communicating situation can be set up with a few symbols that correspond to familiar words. Early movement communications can be tried by having the parents carry out a routine, such as feeding, and helping each parent respond selectively to specific movements. When the children's communications have been accurately assessed and the adaptive system is at the appropriate level, the sampling reactions should be successful. At the conclusion of the evaluation, the children and their parents will have more successful ways to communicate than when the evaluation began. This can be the first step toward a successful intervention process.

INTERVENTION

The intervention model presented here is one which attempts to provide parallel communication strategies whenever normal speech and language skills are not possible for the infant with cerebral palsy (Carlson, 1981). Bloom and Lahey (1978) have proposed a model for language training which includes three components: *content, form,* and *use. Content* refers to the meaning of the message. *Form* refers to the speech sounds, words, and grammatical structure employed. *Use* refers to the purpose of the utterance. When this model is expanded to refer to parallel communication training, the form component is altered and a parallel form is substituted. For example, the movement of signing may be substituted for speech sounds. The form selected must be compatible with the child's motor and perceptual abilities. These parallel or alternate forms of communication can be used to assist the child in acquiring language content (concepts about people, animals, and objects, actions, event processes) and use (knowledge of how and when to use language). The communication partner has the responsibility of recognizing and responding to or creating an environment that will respond to the infant's parallel communication forms.

Ideally, the child with cerebral palsy should have forms of communication at all stages of development and throughout every day that are equivalent to the content and use of their normal peers. For example, the infant unable to phonate voluntarily may substitute a facial expression, general body movement, or gaze response for babbling in a turn-taking social communication. Realistically, it is possible to carry out episodes of parallel communication throughout the day, but difficult if not impossible to do so with the frequency and quality of normal adult-infant interactions.

Reacting to the Child

Didactic teaching does not work with infants. The adult needs to structure situations to which the child can respond. As the adult responds to
the child's reaction, communication and learning occur. Setting up the
situation includes the use of any necessary adaptive equipment, selection
of toys and materials of daily living, and developing procedures which
include the events, sequences, and timing of the communication process.
To some parents, professionals, and community members, this is an instinc-
tive process, and training sessions become a time for encouragement and
reinforcement of good communication skills. In other cases, information,
demonstration, and practice will lead to successful communication and
generalization of those skills to other situations.

Studies of parent-infant interaction have shown that infants initiate,
continue, and terminate communications (Reilly, 1980; Lewis & Rosenblum, 1977). Communicative attempts of the infant with cerebral palsy
are often misinterpreted because of the motor or perceptual problems. As
a result, communications are interrupted, damaged, or ignored. These
infants then either fail entirely or have limited experience in gaining control over their own communications. This may be the reason why so many
older nonspeakers respond to communications initiated by others, but
rarely start conversations (Kraat, 1982; Yoder & Kraat, 1983). Any intervention procedures need to respect the infants' roles as controllers of their
own communication.

Environmental Compensation for Disabilities.   For children with
motor problems, episodes of communicating may need to start with placement in special positions so they can see, feel, or hear the communications (see Chapter 8). The communication partners will also need to place
themselves so that they can be felt, seen, and heard by the child and see,
feel, or hear the child when necessary. For children who are sitting, standing, or lying in special equipment, the listener may need to remember to
maintain tactile contact in order to detect subtle movement communications. When children are held, the listener may need to position a mirror
so that the child's eye movements and facial expression can be read.
Another alternative is to have a second person verify communications not
seen or felt by the first communicator.

Another component of environmental adaptations is the selection of
toys and other materials with which the child can interact. The materials
should be safe as well as cognitively, motorically, and visually appropriate to the child's level of functioning. Many toys and materials can be used
without modification if care is taken to make sure they meet all of the
child's needs. However, this may require invention of a function for a toy
or material that the manufacturer did not originally intend. Normal

infants are inventive in this area. They use shoes as teething rings, spoons as drum sticks, and go through a maddening period of making every object into a ball for throwing. The child with cerebral palsy will be just as inventive whenever possible. One little girl found that glasses were great "take offs" and "bangers," and the velcro fasteners on leg braces were the only things she could "open."

Toys will need to match the child's cognitive and motor abilities. Toys appropriate to a child's cognitive level may be incompatible with the child's motor and perceptual skills. A toy intended for a school age child may be of a size and weight more easily manipulated by the infant with motor problems. Toys for older children tend to be more realistic and may be more appropriate to a handicapped infant's visual needs. Toys made for safe use by age level peers are often too large or difficult for infants with cerebral palsy to manipulate.

Many materials must be adapted before the infant with cerebral palsy can use them. Handles can be attached to items so that they can be grasped. Materials can be suspended on a string so they can be easily moved or be kept accessible. Playboards (devices designed to hold toys for children with cerebral palsy) or other means for attaching items to tables and trays can keep objects within range for manipulation by the infant (Carlson, 1982).

Recently, there has been expanded use of electronic devices controllable by switches designed for operation by children who have cerebral palsy. Switches serve two major functions for these children; they can be used either for environmental control or communication. The same switch or device can potentially be used for both purposes. This poses no problem to the older child who understands the alternating functions of the device, but an infant may not yet make this kind of discrimination.

The type of switch used with infants may be important. One type of switch either stays on or off once it has been activated, like most light switches. The other type stays on only as long as the child continues to maintain switch contact. Either switch appears appropriate for environmental control as an aid to poor motor control because there are normal parallels to both switch activation processes. A single movement can also set off a chain of events or a child can continuously do something to create an event. When communicating, there is a constant action in the form of vocalization, facial expression, or other movement. Only the maintaining switch is comparable to the timing process of communications.

Procedural Compensations for Disabilities. The events, sequences, and timing of any procedure will vary with each child's needs and the process necessary for that particular procedure. Since infancy is the period when rules for the game of communicating are established, there is a need for consistency. Some infants can "pat-a-cake" with Mom and "roughhouse" with Dad, but not vice-versa, because moms and dads do not use recognizable rules for each other's communication game. Intervention involves the process through which both the infant and the parents discover what the rules are. For one infant, Mom and Dad themselves were one of the communication cues. With a little practice, either person in conjunction with specific events became the cue for "pat-a-cake" or "roughhouse." With another infant, the timing was off and with timing repairs, communication occurred with everyone.

Alternate forms of communication often require specific procedural compensations. Compensatory procedures may demand the use of specific materials, certain people, and particular combinations of events or sequences and timing. If any one element is out of synchronization for some children, there is a breakdown in communication. Other children with cerebral palsy can tolerate more flexibility and only a few elements are essential to the process.

Some infants will show a preference for using a more difficult skill. One 2-year-old with an easily executed gaze response insisted on using pointing. In order to point, he had to be seated in a specific chair, the materials needed to be fastened to his tray at a designated spot, and the communication partner had to face him. He would then look at the desired item, pause, throw his arms back, hit at any item, progress through the items until the desired one was reached, pause, sigh, look up at his communication partner, and then expect a response. Even though the partner knew from the first gaze what the child was communicating, he became upset if the process was interrupted.

It is difficult to predict which form of communication infants will use as they grow older. For that reason, children should be introduced to and encouraged to use all possible forms of communicating. Methods of accessing movement, vocal, and visual communication should be presented. If the child resists one form or another, it can be put aside and reintroduced later. The boy in the previous paragraph, for example, used a headstick once he entered elementary school although he resisted when it was introduced earlier.

Children with motor problems often have few situations in which they can make and carry out decisions, no matter how small. Decision making is part of communication and needs to be respected from the beginning. Infants with cerebral palsy often have no interpretable way of letting parents know what they want to wear, play with, or eat. Situations can be created where primitive communications can be interpreted as decisions. For example, parents can hold up clothing items, toys, or foods and clothe, play with, or feed the child whichever one the infant moves or gazes toward.

Because augmentative methods of communication are not standard forms of communicating, infants who are potential nonspeakers are not exposed to the form of communication they will use. Infants who will speak, hear speech from the beginning. When motorically and cognitively ready to begin talking, they have experiences with spoken language. If parents and other community members use augmentative methods to communicate with infants who potentially need it, their experiences will parallel normal. The child will observe how the system operates and come to recognize its value.

Reacting to the Child's Expressive Communication Abilities.

Learning to communicate in standard forms goes beyond exposure to those forms. Parents selectively respond to infant behaviors which resemble adult communications. In order to parallel normal communication, parents of children with cerebral palsy may need to respond to any of the infant's behaviors which have potential for communication. The child then learns that movement, eye gaze, and sound making are forms of communicating. If and when the child's systems mature, they can be refined.

Infants with cerebral palsy often have early behaviors that are subtle, exaggerated, or aberrant. If these are the only behaviors available to the child, they are the only ones the infant can use to communicate. Before it becomes a communication, the behavior must consistently be combined with the appropriate event. For example, one little girl retracted her foot when her shoe touched the foot in dressing and went through exaggerated smacking movements after she had swallowed a bite of food. The mother treated the movements as signals for dressing and eating although they were unintentional. In time, the little girl used them purposefully. She used them to initiate communications as well as to respond to others.

As motor skills improve, more sophisticated communications are possible. Infants with experience as communicators will often demonstrate readiness to move to the next step on their own. The little girl mentioned previously began to invent gestures as her hand skills improved. She would repeat the same gesture over and over until the adult figured out the meaning.

Some children do not move on to new communication forms easily. Instructing community members to respond to the primitive response more slowly and with less accuracy than the more mature communications has been an effective technique. Many children use the crying response long after they have other vocal forms of communication. One little boy persisted in using a cry after he had gained voluntary control over a few phonations. He did not appear to realize that he could call someone in any other way. His family began to treat his accidental phonations as "words" and gave him immediate and appropriate attention. When he cried, they checked to see if he was in distress, and if not, delayed responding or responded inappropriately even though they had read his intent. He soon discovered that phonating was an effective form of communication and reduced the crying.

Successful communication may drop out in one or all situations if others do not respond to the child's self-initiated communications. Spontaneous initiation of gestures stopped at home in the case of the little girl mentioned earlier when she entered a preschool with a more directive approach. For example, communication centered around activities where she was requested "tell me . . ." or "show teacher . . ." rather than waiting for self-initiated communication within play situations. As the approach was changed, the little girl again spontaneously gestured.

Documenting Communication Abilities. Many of the communications used by infants with cerebral palsy are not familiar or easily recognized as communication behaviors. By describing and documenting these behaviors, they can be treated as communication by anyone interacting with the child. This can be done in the form of a "Communication Dictionary" (Carlson, 1981). The dictionary can take the form of a poster, a notebook, or a diary. Each behavior can be described or illustrated and the corresponding intent or meaning would be listed.

Parent Training

Parent training includes the instruction of anyone who routinely interacts with the child. Often siblings or other children communicate more effectively with the infant who has cerebral palsy and benefit from training more than adults do.

The problems of severely involved children are many, and sometimes caretakers are so overwhelmed by the difficulties of caregiving that it is hard to remember to use specialized communications. Care must be taken to devise and employ communication strategies which fit into or accommodate the physiological needs of the child. Communication strategies that do not mesh with the routine of care and the needs of the child and family will not be carried out with sufficient frequency to be effective.

Education. To educate parents, clinicians need to be knowledgeable about cerebral palsy and its effect on communication in infants. They should be able to explain why each evaluation procedure is conducted and what the implications of the results are for communication intervention. Some children, however, have unique problems and many of the nonspeech strategies are so new that there is not sufficient background for a broad knowledge base. Honesty in education is the best policy in these cases. It is generally good practice to explain to parents that they and their child are pioneers in the communication strategies being utilized and explain to them the philosophies behind the intervention techniques. With this type of education, many parents become good problem solvers. Rather than giving the parents a set of techniques to use, the clinician has given the parents a way to create their own solutions. The techniques and strategies developed by parents are often more functional in the family situation than those developed by clinicians.

Training should include information about materials, devices, and systems that may be potentially helpful to their child. Parents may need information regarding funding sources, available services, and the rights of handicapped children and their families.

Parents have differing capacities for the level, amount, and rate at which they can handle educational information. The speech-language pathologist should have an awareness of the parents' abilities and learning styles during training. An open atmosphere should encourage parents to communicate freely their problems, successes, and needs to the clinician.

Facilitation.   With some parents, the previously described education is all the parent training that is necessary. The training process then becomes one of updating them as their child matures or new information and materials become available. With other parents, direct intervention, demonstration, and practice are needed to facilitate the training process. Many of the strategies involve unique ways of communication that are often difficult for families to generalize to new situations and much repetition is necessary.

With young or more severely handicapped infants, the environment in which communication occurs may be a component of the communication act. In these cases, training is more functional when it takes place in the home or other places where the communication actually occurs. Sometimes it is possible to simulate within the therapy room an environment that cannot be visited.

Sometimes it may be necessary to abandon long-range goals for a period in order to meet special needs such as communication during hospitalization for tests or surgery. The mother of one child expressed the fear that her child's limited symbol and gesture communication would be inadequate for a hospital stay. The mother was instructed in how to communicate with her child through play and demonstration using a doll as well as real and toy medical instruments. These same materials were sent with the mother and child when they went to the hospital. The child tolerated well all tests where play demonstration and communication was permitted.

Encouragement.   Many parents have training or skills applicable to their child's needs. In these cases, training will take the form of encouraging the parents to begin or to continue to apply their knowledge to the child's needs.

Sometimes, the parent may have more background in some of the child's need areas than the speech-language pathologist. For example, a father with a background in electronics may know more about how electronic communication devices function than most speech-language pathologists. Parents should be encouraged to share that knowledge.

EMERGING FROM INFANCY

As children emerge from infancy, they are beginning to use symbolic forms of communication—speech, visual symbols, signs, or a combination of systems. The early strategies will have formed a foundation for these more advanced forms.

Foundations for Speech

Early responses to vocalizations should let children know that they can have a measure of control over their world by the sounds they make. At a minimum, the child can use vocalization as a signal call. The more skilled child will have used even aberrant patterns as speech approximations that may in time become more intelligible speech.

Foundations for Alternate Communication

If speech develops, the alternate communication will drop out, but it will have served its purpose for a time. If speech does not develop, the child can look forward to more sophisticated signing, using electronic communication devices, and symbols for communicating.

Helping Parents Look Ahead

Some parents verbalize their apprehensions about the future, others do not, but remain concerned. The speech-language pathologist will need to make the parents aware of the unfamiliar steps in alternate communication or adapted speech development. Parents need to know that augmentative communication is a relatively new field, and as a result, predictions for the future are guesses at best. Fortunately, recent developments make the promise of effective communication beyond infancy brighter than in the past.

REFERENCES

Bloom, L., & Lahey, M. (1978). *Language development and language disorders.* New York: John Wiley & Sons.

Bzoch, K., & League, R. (1971). *Receptive-Expressive Emergent Language Scale.* Austin, TX: PRO-ED.

Carlson, F. (1981). *Alternate methods of communication.* Danville, IL: The Interstate Printers and Publishers.

Carlson, F. (1982). *Prattle and play.* Omaha, NE: Meyer Children's Rehabilitation Institute Media Resource Center.

George, C. (1983). *Sensorimotor communication profile.* Paper presented at Meyer Children's Rehabilitation Institute, University of Nebraska Medical Center, Omaha, NE.

Hedrick, D. L., Prather, E. M., & Tobin, A. R. (1975). *Sequenced inventory of communication development.* Seattle, WA: University of Washington Press.

Kraat, A. (1982, January). *Issues in the application of augmentative communication . . . social, training, measurement.* Paper presented at Communication Problems in Children Series, Omaha, NE.

Lewis, M., & Rosenblum, L. A. (Eds.). (1977). *Interaction, conversation, and development of language.* New York: John Wiley & Sons.

Piaget, J. (1952). *The origins of intelligence in children.* New York: Basic Books.

Piaget, J., & Inhelder, B. (1969). *The psychology of the child.* New York: Basic Books.

Reilly, A. P. (Ed.). (1980). *The communication game,* 4, Johnson & Johnson Baby Products Company Pediatric Round Table Series.

Shane, H. C., & Bashir, A. S. (1980). Election criteria for the adoption of an augmentative communication system: Preliminary considerations. *Journal of Speech and Hearing Disorders, 45,* 408–414.

Silverman, F. H. (1980). *Communication for the speechless.* Englewood Cliffs, NJ: Prentice-Hall.

Wasson, P., Tynan, T., & Gardiner, P. (1982). *Test adaptations for the handicapped.* San Antonio, TX: Educational Service Center Region 20.

Ylvisaker, M. (1981). *Assessment of infant communication development: A new approach.* Paper presented at The Rehabilitation Institute of Pittsburgh, Pittsburgh, PA.

Yoder, D. E., & Kraat, A. (1983). Intervention issues in nonspeech communication. In J. Miller, D. Yoder, & R. Schiefelbusch (Eds.), *Contemporary issues in language intervention,* (pp. 27–52). AHSA Report #12.

CHAPTER 11

Augmentative Communication

Caroline R. Musselwhite

> *Musselwhite suggests that a systematic process of decision making, consisting of several stages, should be followed when considering, developing, and implementing an augmentative communication program. Many symbol systems are now available. They may be displayed in a variety of formats and accessed in different ways, depending on the capabilities of the user. Users must be taught how to communicate with an aid and strategies developed to enhance communicative interactions between the cerebral palsied individuals and other persons.*

1. *For each stage in the decision making process, list (a) the factors to be considered, and (b) the decisions which might be made.*
2. *List and describe the symbol systems discussed and indicate for each the sources (see References) of additional information about the system.*
3. *What factors should be considered in selecting (a) the symbol system, and (b) a method of indicating symbols selected for a message?*
4. *What strategies might you use to overcome the barriers to effective communication between an aided speaker and a natural speaker?*

GENERAL CONSIDERATIONS

It would not be possible to overstate the importance of communication for cognitive and social-emotional development. Some persons with cerebral palsy cannot learn to communicate effectively by means of speech because of their neuromuscular dysfunction. As a group, they are often referred to as "nonspeaking" (ASHA Ad Hoc Committee on Communication Processes and Nonspeaking Persons, 1981). This label is, in part, a misnomer because many in the group do produce some speech; however, their intelligibility is inadequate for communication. For convenience, however, the terms *nonspeaking* and *nonspeaker* will be used in this chapter to mean those who produce little or no speech, and those whose speech is of low intelligibility. For all these persons, it is imperative that they be taught another mode of expression to augment their communicative efforts.

Between the first suggestion that an augmentative communication system might be appropriate and the actual implementation of a system, a series of increasingly fine decisions must be made. This decision process must be ongoing. Not only must it address existing concerns (e.g., frequent communication breakdowns) but it must meet new challenges (e.g., mainstreaming into a scout troop). Whether this decision making process is structured or haphazard, crucial decisions are constantly being made.

A four-stage structured approach to decision making is outlined in this chapter. Strategies designed to bring this decision process to a high level of awareness are discussed and procedures are described for making choices based on the best available information regarding augmentative communication in general as well as the specific needs and abilities of the nonspeaker.

STAGE I:
THE SPEECH/NONSPEECH DECISION

This initial decision is often termed the *election decision* (Blau, 1983; Shane, 1981) because it involves the decision to implement an augmentative communication system. The branching-type decision matrix developed by Shane and Bashir (1980) structures the election process so that crucial features are not ignored. Their matrix considers the factors presented in Table 11.1 and is useful in identifying children at risk for speech development. A high risk child who is not yet ready for a formal augmentative communication may be a candidate for early nonspeech oriented activities such as those discussed by Carlson in Chapter 10 and Musselwhite and St. Louis (1982).

TABLE 11.1
Factors Indicating the Need for an
Augmentative Communication System

FACTORS & EXAMPLES	KEY POINTS TO CONSIDER
Cognitive Factors MA of 18 months	Stage V of sensorimotor development appears necessary for conventional communication (speech, symbols)
Oral Reflex Factors rooting, bite	Especially powerful; presence in isolation can yield election decision; predictive of oral speech failure
Language & Motor Speech Production Factors receptive/expressive discrepancy	Consider intervening with augmentative communication before the gap becomes too large; avoid frustration
Motor Speech: Contributing Factors eating problems, apraxia, drooling	Research has related these factors to difficulty or failure in oral speech
Production: Contributing Factors unintelligible speech, frustration	Taken together, these factors can suggest that oral speech alone is inadequate
Emotional Factors selective mutism	Children selectively withholding speech may have better success using augmentative communication
Chronological Age Factors under 3? over 5?	Formal systems not productive until 18 months, but may begin informal introduction earlier
Previous Therapy Factors appropriateness; progress too slow	Appropriate but ineffective prespeech/speech therapy suggests need for intervention with augmentative approaches
Previous Therapy: Contributing Factors motor, oral, vocal imitation	Nonimitative children are less likely to be successful in vocal instruction
Implementation Factors: Environment family acceptance	Lack of parental support will sabotage success (see Musselwhite & St. Louis, 1982 for suggestions)

Adapted from Shane (1981) and Shane and Bashir (1980).

The decision to initiate an augmentative system should not be interpreted as meaning that speech will not develop or that no effort will be made to help the child develop speech. While there are many nonspeakers for whom nonspeech systems serve a *primary* function, Harris and Vanderheiden (1980) stress that these techniques ". . . be viewed as *augmentative* or supplementary techniques that enhance communication by complementing whatever vocal skills the individual may possess" (p. 233). When viewed from this perspective, the decision may be seen as one of emphasis, rather than strictly an either/or choice. Nonspeech systems have been found to *facilitate* the development of both communication and speech skills (Silverman, 1980). Nonspeech systems can also be *supplemental*, used only in certain situations—when communicating with unfamiliar listeners or when pronunciation of a word is not intelligible.

To summarize, the decision to elect a nonspeech system can have a powerful impact on the nonspeaker and on his or her communication partners. It is important that the team make a carefully considered decision rather than initiate an augmentative system because this procedure is currently popular, or ignore other augmentative techniques due to lack of knowledge about them.

STAGE II:
THE AIDED/UNAIDED DECISION

After deciding to use an augmentative system, the team must next decide whether teaching should use an aided or unaided system. *Aided* refers to ". . . all techniques where some type of physical object or device is used," while *unaided* refers to ". . . all techniques which do not require any physical aids" (ASHA Ad Hoc Committee on Communication Processes and Nonspeaking Persons, 1981, p. 578).

In practice the choice between aided and unaided is often determined by the nature of the child's disability. Kiernan, Reid, and Jones (1979) found that schools for the mentally retarded favored the use of signs, while schools for the physically handicapped preferred symbol use. Although the possibility of successful signing may be ruled out for some people with severe motor disabilities, the use of gross movements codified into an unaided system is an option for many moderately involved nonspeakers.

It is unlikely that an unaided system alone could provide a nonspeaker with cerebral palsy sufficient speed, ease of communication, and available audience. However, it might provide a needed supplement to an aided system, in selected *situations* (e.g., when a communication device is unavailable or not working), with certain *communication partners* (e.g., parents and siblings, who have learned the signs), and for *communication at a distance* (e.g., across a room). As Shane (1981) notes, it may not be feasible to provide equal training time for two separate systems; thus one system, such as Blissymbolics, may be trained formally, while another, for example Duffy's System, may be informally introduced.

STAGE III:
SYSTEM SELECTION

There are many systems, aided and unaided, through which nonspeaking persons may express themselves. The system selected and the vocabulary available affect the user's success in communicating (Yoder & Kraat, 1983).

Unaided System

As noted previously, some nonspeakers with cerebral palsy will be able to use unaided, or gestural systems, at least for supplemental communication while the motoric requirements for most unaided systems (e.g., American Sign Language, Signed English, fingerspelling) are too demanding for many nonspeakers with cerebral palsy. Several systems may be useable, either in traditional or adapted form.

Duffy's System. This logically based system was developed by a special education teacher working with four quadriplegic cerebral palsied students (Duffy, 1977). It includes 471 signs formed by gross gestures such as raising an arm or placing a hand on the knee. Some signs are accompanied by vocalizations (primarily vowels) to encourage vocal output. Signs within a category, such as days of the week, are typically preceded by a general category sign. For example, SUNDAY is signed by combining the signs for DAY and ONE, since SUNDAY is the first day of the week. Alphanumeric entries are included. Thus, a small number of basic movements yields nearly 500 signs, making this system feasible for people with limited gross motor control. Clearly, rate of output would be reduced, with two or more gestures needed to encode a single concept such as SUNDAY. In summary, Duffy's System could be highly productive when used in a closed environment (e.g., with family members) at times when an aided system is not desired or not available.

Amer-Ind. Amer-Ind (Skelly, 1979) is a signal system based on American Indian Hand Talk. It is nonlinguistic, meaning that it is not based on any spoken or written language. It is highly action oriented, with signals representing broad concepts which in turn suggest specific words. The 250 concept labels (e.g., *quiet*) represent approximately 2500 English word equivalents, but specific meaning of a signal is flexible, depending on context. Amer-Ind has potential as a supplemental system for persons having adequate control of one arm, as 80% of the signal repertoire can be executed with one hand, and the remaining signals can be adapted for one-handed use or substituted. Daniloff, Lloyd, and Fristoe (1983) found that Amer-Ind is 42–50% transparent, or guessable, in its citation form and note that this is significantly more transparent than the 10–30% levels reported for American Sign Language by Hoemann (1975). They also suggest that actual transparency levels could be enhanced slightly when the signals are produced in context, due to the addition of situational cues. Thus, Amer-Ind could provide a moderately transparent system to supplement aided communication.

Idiosyncratic Signals. Supplemental gestures should be considered for all nonspeakers using aided systems since, by definition, aided systems require access to symbols extraneous to the body. Thus, there will be times, such as bathing, toileting, or during physical therapy, when aided systems will be unavailable. At a minimum, nonspeakers should be able to directly signal *yes, no,* and *get my board.*

Some nonspeakers can build a repertoire of usable signals from gross movements similar to those included in Duffy's System. Bottorf and DePape (1982) suggest the following criteria for selecting communication signals: ease and speed of production, minimal fatigue, ease of recognition by partners, and low frequency of involuntary movements that could be confused with signals. These idiosyncratic signals, as well as conventional signs, should be described on a Communication Report Form such as the one presented by Kollinzas (1983), so that all potential communication partners can interpret them.

Aided Systems

Aided, or symbolic, systems can be categorized (Musselwhite & St. Louis, 1982) based on features of origin, type, and intent. The chapter will focus on representational systems and symbolic language codes, as they are most often used on communication displays (Kiernan et al., 1979).

Representational Symbol Systems. A wide range of symbols can be found within this category, from highly concrete (e.g., an actual object) to relatively obscure representations (e.g., a combination of the Blissymbols for mind ⌒ and enclosure ☐ to indicate knowledge ⌂). As a group, representational systems include primarily symbols that are *pictographic* (picture what they represent) or *ideographic* (depict ideas about the referent). Representational systems have relatively few symbols that are *arbitrary* (having meaning assigned, but not suggested by the symbol). Figure 11.1 illustrates symbols of each type from several widely used representational systems. Primary references for obtaining further information on each system are also provided.

Blissymbolics. Blissymbolics is a graphic nonalphabet communication system, originally intended to serve as an internal communication medium (McNaughton & Kates, 1980). It was developed by Charles K. Bliss over a period of more than 20 years, and has been used by physically impaired, nonspeaking people since 1971.

Over 1400 different Blissymbols are presented in *Blissymbols for Use* (Hehner, 1980). These symbols represent combinations, or agglutinations, of 100 basic symbol elements (e.g., circle, slash, pointer). Through a variety of expansion techniques, a much larger number of words can be represented (McDonald, 1980a). The meaning of a Blissymbol can be altered by slight changes in features such as size, position, and spacing of symbol elements. Several Blissymbol *indicators* (Figure 11.2) can be added to code grammatical information (plurality, verb tense, or part of speech). Several *strategies* (Figure 11.2) can also enlarge the possible Blissymbol vocabulary. Any user or instructor may create a new, "combined" symbol, for personal use only, if a standard symbol is not available. Because the entire system is based on approximately 100 basic elements, symbols can be easily reproduced, enlarged, or reduced by hand, with the aid of a template or grid.

McNaughton and Kates (1980) report that "Blissymbolics has been demonstrated as particularly valuable to physically handicapped persons whose physical limitations restrict them to a specific number of symbols" (p. 311). This is due to the extensive combinational features described previously. The Blissymbolics Communication Institute (BCI) in Toronto has been developed to provide support to Blissymbol users and instructors, and to their communication partners. Training sessions and a wide variety of texts, materials, and other information on Blissymbolics are available through BCI.

Picsyms. Picsyms (Carlson, 1981b) is a graphic system based on the language of young children and designed specifically for communication interchange with prereaders. It follows highly logical principles, yielding an open-ended system so that users and instructors can create new symbols following a set of guidelines. The system is still under development; when completed, it will include 1800 symbol-words.

Picsyms uses the technique of agglutination, combining symbol elements to form new symbols. However, this is accomplished within one "frame" or box, such that a single symbol represents each referent. For example, each of the seven Picsyms illustrated in Figure 11.2 would be enclosed in a real or imaginary box on a communication display. A variety of tactics can be used to indicate changes in meaning for basic symbol elements, as illustrated in Figure 11.2. Picsyms are readily reproduced, enlarged, or reduced by hand, using a grid or a template.

Developmental or maturational variations, such as adding details to symbols when necessary, are included to make the system adaptable to a wide receptive language range. Some abstract concepts (e.g., conjunc-

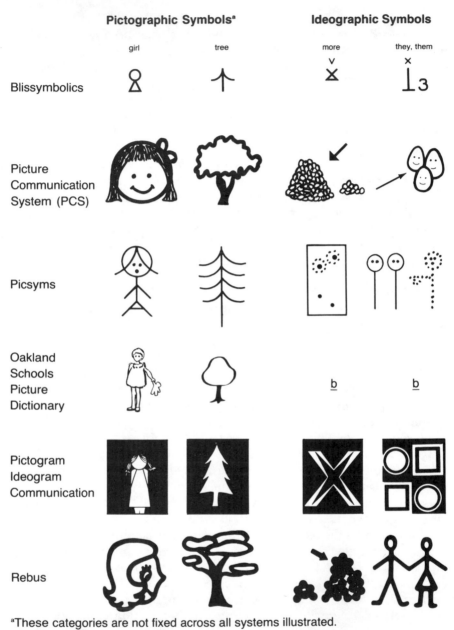

Figure 11.1. Representational symbol systems.

Arbitrary Symbols	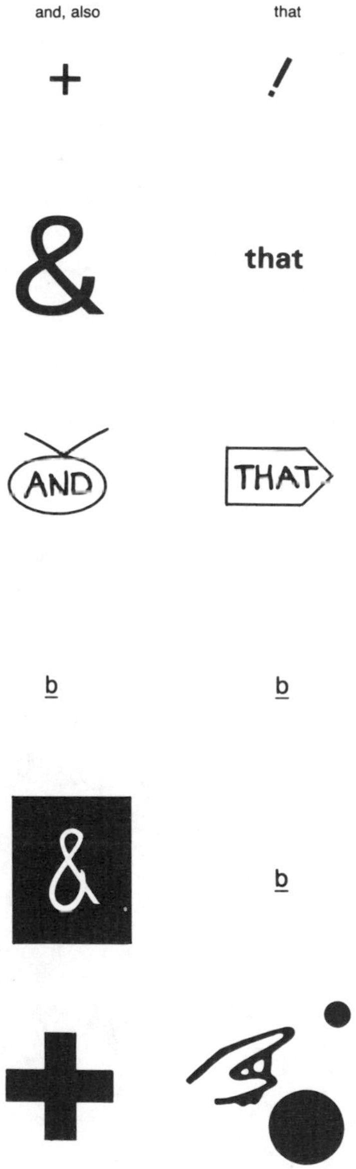	**Primary Resources**
and, also	that	
+	*!*	Blissymbolics Communication Institute 350 Rumsey Road Toronto, Ontario, Canada M4G 1R8
&	**that**	Mayer-Johnson Company P.O. Box AD Solana Beach, CA 92075
(AND)	THAT	Baggeboda Press 1128 Rhode Island St. Lawrence, KS 66044
b	b	Oakland Schools 2100 Pontiac Lake Road Pontiac, MI 48054
&	b	George Reed Foundation Box 1547 Regina, Saskatchewan S4P 3C4
+		American Guidance Service Publishers Building Circle Pines, MN 55014

Figure 11.1. Continued.

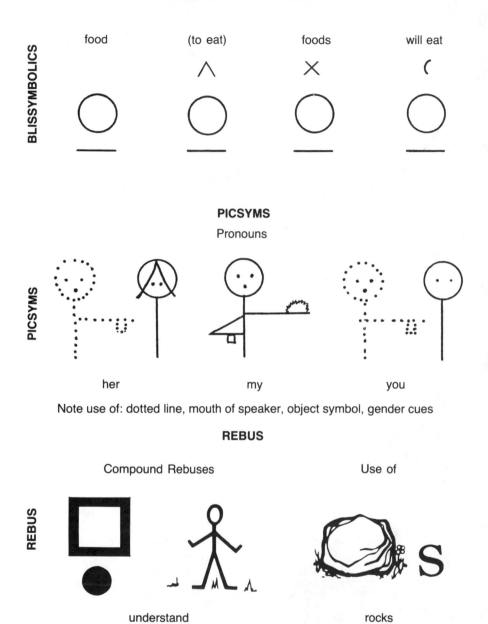

BLISSYMBOL INDICATORS

BLISSYMBOLICS

food   (to eat)   foods   will eat

PICSYMS
Pronouns

PICSYMS

her   my   you

Note use of: dotted line, mouth of speaker, object symbol, gender cues

REBUS

Compound Rebuses   Use of

REBUS

understand   rocks

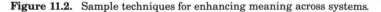

Figure 11.2. Sample techniques for enhancing meaning across systems.

BLISSYMBOL STRATEGIES

cold   drop   loud

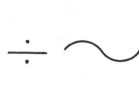   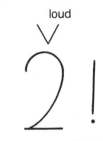

(opposite of hot)   (part of water)   (sound intensified)

TACTICS

Noun-Verb Pairs   Time

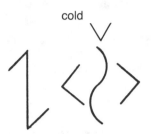

snow (noun)   snow (verb)   today

Note use of directional arrows   tomorrow

Note use of dot

COMBINATIONS

Affixes   Use of letters

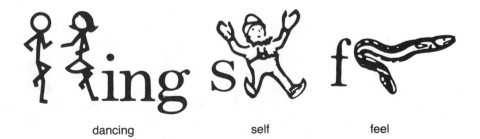

dancing   self   feel

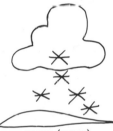

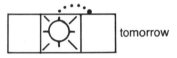

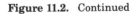

Figure 11.2. Continued

tions) are represented by combining traditional orthography with a general symbol (Figure 11.1) to allow eventual fading of symbols to words.

Rebus.   Rebuses are symbols that represent an entire word or part of a word. The *Standard Rebus Glossary* (Clark, Davies, & Woodcock, 1974) includes 818 different rebuses, with combinations yielding representation of more than 2000 words. This set of rebuses was initially designed to aid in teaching reading. Users may design additional rebus symbols as needed.

Rebuses are typically pictographic (Figures 11.1 and 11.2). It is, to some extent, a phonetically-based system, with many pictographs related to their referents through sound rather than meaning. For example, pictographs for BEE, WOOD, and TWO (2) represent the words "be," "would," and "to/too." Several combinations of rebuses, or rebuses plus traditional orthography serve to expand the rebus vocabulary. The symbols for HELPING, BUSES, DRAIN, and PINCH illustrate this procedure (Figure 11.2).

Rebuses are available in rub-on form or on rebus cards. Many rebuses are difficult to reproduce accurately by hand. Materials designed for implementation of rebus symbols by disabled persons are available (see Figure 11.1 for source).

Other Commercially Available Symbol Sets.   Three additional symbol sets are described briefly and illustrated in Figure 11.1. The *Picture Communication Symbols* (PCS) consist primarily of over 1800 simple line drawings that may be reproduced by photocopying. They are available in 1- and 2-inch sizes that are organized by categories in two binders. A guide booklet suggesting implementation strategies is included.

The *Oakland School's Picture Dictionary*, developed by Ina Kirstein, contains over 500 simple line drawings divided into 20 categories with alphabetical and categorical indexes. Three sizes of drawings are included: 2-inch, 1-inch, and ½-inch. They are intended to serve as a bridge between photographs and symbol systems.

The *Pictograph Ideogram Communication* (PIC) set includes 400 symbols available in two sizes (2 in. x 2 in. and 5/8 in. x 7/8 in). Unlike most systems, symbols are white on a black background. Anecdotal reports suggest that this is helpful for people with visual-perceptual problems, but research is needed to investigate this theory. Some symbols include considerable detail while others are highly stylized. Programming materials include specific assessment and training components and data sheets.

Symbolic Language Codes.   This category encompasses systems that represent a spoken or written language. Several subcategories may be useful for nonspeakers having cerebral palsy.

Alphabetic Representations.   The alphabet may be presented in several formats. Use of an *alphabet board* ranges from spelling entire words to *initial letter cueing*, or pointing to the first letter of each word as an attempt is made to vocalize the word. Beukelman and Yorkston (1982) examined rate of expression in acquired dysarthric speakers and found an average rate of 28 words per minute when spelling entire words. Letters can also be *chunked*, based on frequency of occurrence in English, as in the WRITE system (Goodenough-Trepagnier, Tarry, & Prather, 1982). Chunking refers to combining frequently occurring letter sequences; the purpose is to reduce the number of selections needed to communicate a word. Inclusion of an alphabet within the display allows production of an unlimited vocabulary. Communication displays may also include *words or phrases*; these will increase rate of expression, but available vocabulary will be limited unless the alphabet is included. Displays often include a combination of these formats to enhance both rate and size of vocabulary.

Phonemic Representations. As Goodenough-Trepagnier and Prather (1981) point out, sound-based systems are more economical than spelling-based systems because English sounds may be represented in such varied ways through traditional orthography. In addition, a sound-based system can ignore silent letters and can use one symbol rather than two to indicate a diagraph such as "sh." It is also suggested that a sound-based system would be easier for nonreaders to learn.

The SPEEC system has been developed to increase speed of expression by chunking sounds, as the WRITE system chunks letters. Two versions of SPEEC are available, one of 256 and the other of 400 units. Each presents the units in two arrangements—one, a traditional alphabetic arrangement, and the other according to frequency of occurrence in speech. Goodenough-Trepagnier and Prather (1981), developers of the system, report that letter-by-letter spelling requires 2.44 times as many selection gestures as SPEEC-400. An example will suggest the organization and efficiency of the SPEEC system: The chunk of sounds SUHN is included because it occurs frequently in words (son, sun), and as part of words (Sunday, person, messenger). A SPEEC manual is available to aid in implementing the system (Goodenough-Trepagnier & Prather, 1979).

The sound-based Cued Speech system (Henegar & Cornett, 1981) has been adapted as a visual system by Clark (1984) and is termed *NUE-VUE-CUE™*. This system uses a plexiglass E-tran type board with consonant sounds (indicated by hand cues and letters) placed at the eight points of a Tic-Tac-Toe arrangement, and vowels and diphthongs placed at the outer corners, as illustrated in Figure 11.3. Color codes on the inside edges are used to represent mouth configurations (e.g., bilabial, tip-alveolar). Words can then be built by combining sound chunks. For example, "teachers" is formed by indicating T + E + CH + UR + Z. Since the chart includes only eight hand configurations, five vowel/diphthong sets, and five colors, use of eye gaze is feasible for many nonspeakers. NU-VUE-CUE has been used successfully with children as young as 5 years of age (Roselyn Clark, personal communication).

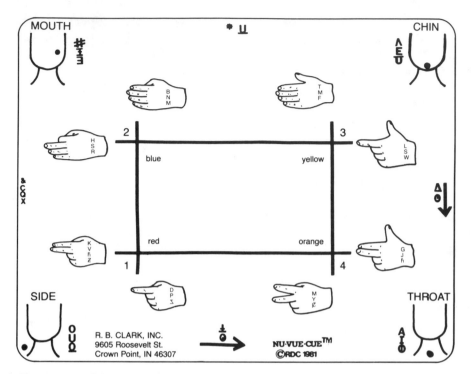

Figure 11.3. Schematic of NU-VUE-CUE™ chart.

Encoded Alphabetic Representations. The *International Morse Code* represents the letters of the Roman alphabet. In Morse Code, letters, digits, and several additional elements are indicated through a series of dots and dashes. For nonspeaking persons, these can be coded directly (e.g., by using a switch), by indicating symbols for dot and dash, or by using gestures (e.g., short blink = dot, long blink = dash). The American Radio Relay League (225 Main Street, Newington, CT 05111) can provide materials for learning and teaching Morse Code, as well as addresses of licensed instructors.

Factors to Consider in System Selection

Following are several criteria to be considered in choosing the primary nonspeech system (Lloyd, 1982; Musselwhite, 1982). The emphasis placed on each will vary with the individual nonspeaker.

Intelligibility. This refers to the ease with which symbols or gestures can be identified without additional cues such as printed words or verbal prompts. It is similar to the concept of transparency, or guessability, of signs or symbols. Symbol intelligibility is important to both the nonspeaker and the communication partners. For example, Musselwhite and Ruscello (1984) found that both Picsyms and Rebus symbols were significantly easier to guess than were Blissymbols for four age groups (ranging from 3 years to 21 years). This was especially notable for subjects under age 6 years, 11 months; those subject groups achieved only random scores for Blissymbolics on a closed-choice format symbol test. This factor is even more important for unaided systems, as printed labels do not accompany gestures. Refer, for example, to the transparency differences between Amer-Ind and ASL, presented earlier.

Ease of Acquisition. In general, research has suggested that representational symbol systems (e.g., Blissymbolics, Picsyms, Rebus) are more readily learned than abstract systems (e.g., Carrier-Peak type symbols, masonite shapes that do not depict the referent), which in turn are more easily acquired than symbolic language codes. Musselwhite (1982) provides a review of this literature.

Correspondence to Community Language. This factor reflects the extent to which systems are used in the community, or can be made to correspond to spoken language. Some unaided systems (e.g., Signing Exact English) more closely parallel the structure of spoken English than do others (e.g., Amer-Ind). Similarly, extensive aided systems such Blissymbolics can parallel spoken or written English more than limited systems such as PIC.

Flexibility. This encompasses several subfactors, each of which contributes to the flexibility of a system. The available *vocabulary size*, and the *utility of the vocabulary* influence the specificity of message production. Blissymbolics, Picsyms, and Rebus all include representations for more than 1500 words. However, comparison of these symbol systems to the 1000 words of *A Spoken Word Count* (Jones & Wepman, 1966) revealed that, for 6 of the 12 grammatical categories, Rebus counts of words represented were at least 10% below those for Blissymbolics and Picsyms (Musselwhite, 1982). A review of the *Standard Rebus Glossary* Clark et al., 1974) suggests that many Rebus symbols may be chosen more for their ability to be pictured than for their potential usefulness. For example, 53 compound symbols are formed with "over"; many of these (e.g., overbear, overfish, overskirt) are minimally functional.

A related issue is the *expansion capability* of a system. This is unlimited for traditional orthography and extensive for both Blissymbolics (through use of strategies and combining) and Picsyms (through use of tactics and guidelines for creating new symbols).

The *adaptability* of a system may be crucial for potential users. Amer-Ind is motorically adaptable, as most signals are or can be one-handed. Picsyms and Blissymbols are examples of visually adaptable systems, as elements can be added to make symbols more meaningful to individual users.

The *ease of symbol reproduction* is another component of flexibility. This involves the simplicity in reproducing symbols in terms of accuracy, time, cost, spontaneity, and output type. Blissymbolics, Picsyms, and symbolic language codes such as the alphabet share advantages of this feature, as they can be readily and inexpensively prepared by hand, with or without the use of a template. These systems are also most amenable to computer and printed output.

Acceptability. This factor is of prime importance to user motivation and partner interaction, but few data are available. Traditional orthography and pictures would be expected to have ready acceptance, since they are quite normative. However, this is a highly individual decision, which may be influenced by exposure to a system. Beukelman and Yorkston (1982) suggest that age may influence perceived acceptability; for example, adults may not tolerate restricted systems that children readily accept.

Efficiency. This factor is related to the number of entries required to yield a sufficient vocabulary and the number of movements necessary to indicate a word. A trade-off may be necessary. For example, systems using agglutination (e.g., Amer-Ind, Blissymbolics, the alphabet) may require fewer entries but more movements to produce a message. Several systems described previously (SPEEC, WRITE, NU-VUE-CUE™) are attempts to compromise between the number of entries and the number of movements required to yield the maximum possible vocabulary with the minimum possible effort. Electronic devices such as Minspeak (Baker, 1983) have also been designed to address the issue of efficiency.

The six criteria described above are factors inherent in the various aided and unaided systems; they are not mutually exclusive, but interact with each other. The cognitive level, motoric skills, and communication environment of the individual nonspeaker must be determined to rule out inappropriate systems. Then the constellation of needs, preferences, and abilities of the nonspeaker must be considered to make the optimal match between system and user.

STAGE IV: SYSTEM IMPLEMENTATION

Successful utilization of an augmentative communication system can be enhanced or obstructed, depending on the decisions made regarding implementation. Primary focus will be on implementation of nonelectronic devices, as electronic devices are discussed in Chapter 13 of this book.

Accessing the System

Three general methods of indicating elements (letters, words, symbols) selected for a message are described in Table 11.2. A number of factors must be considered in choosing one or a combination of these methods:

TABLE 11.2
Means of Indicating Message Elements[a]

METHOD	DESCRIPTION	EXAMPLES
DIRECT SELECTION	User indicates message elements by pointing directly to them	Unaided body part (hand, foot) Appliances (headstick, mouthstick, sliding pointer)
SCANNING	Message elements are presented one at a time; user indicates desired element	Twenty questions Electronic devices (rotary, direct, row-column scanner)
ENCODING	Pattern or code of signals to indicate message elements	Two-movement encoding -two numbers (21 = help) -number + color Morse Code
COMBINATIONS	Desirable features of two techniques are combined	Pointing to large numbers for encoding Point to area, then scan for target entry

[a]For further information, see Harris and Vanderheiden (1980); A Guide to Controls (1982).

1. *Accuracy:* While pointing directly with a hand is more conventional, pointing with a mouthstick or encoding might allow smaller symbols to be indicated with fewer errors.
2. *Speed:* Speed of indicating contributes to output rate and must be optimized to increase the potential for successful interactions.
3. *Effort:* A high degree of effort will slow the rate and contribute to fatigue.
4. *Cognitive demands:* Scanning and encoding require greater cognitive demands than direct selection.
5. *Listener demands:* The effort required of the communication partner (e.g., learning the coding system, verifying responses) may determine whether the user is free to communicate with a large number of partners or limited to those willing or able to interpret the message.

There is a potential for interaction among these factors. For example, an apparent increase in speed through direct selection could result in a reduction in accuracy and, consequently, an actual decrease in rate, due to miscommunications.

Direct selection, scanning, encoding, or combinations of these may be used when pointing by hand or eye, or when using electro-mechanical communication devices.

Developing an Eye Pointing Response. For severely physically disabled nonspeakers, eye pointing can be highly effective as an initial means of indicating, as a method of accessing encoded systems, or as a back-up when electronic devices are unavailable or not working. Warrick (1982) notes that use of eye gaze for direct selection is highly limiting, while *encoding* through eye pointing can be quite rapid and powerful. One example of encoding through eye pointing makes use of a "row-column" or "X-Y" code (McDonald, 1980b). In this arrangement, each row and each column is designated in some way. For example, rows could be indicated by colors and columns by numerals. (For younger children, shapes or pictures of animals could be substituted for the colors or numerals). The colors and numerals are also placed around the perimeter of the display or on a separate board, so the nonspeaker can eye point first to the color (to select the desired row), then to the numeral (to choose the desired column).

Another approach, *quartering*, relates blocks of squares on the communication display to the four corners of an interface frame; this frame is typically a large plexiglass rectangle with the center cut out to allow the nonspeaker to look through it. The user divides the display into four quarters by successive eye pointing to one corner of the frame. For example, a gaze to the upper left corner of the interface frame would indicate that the target entry is located in the upper left block of the display. Successive eye pointing can divide that block into four smaller blocks, and so on. Encoding and quartering can be combined by placing colors and/or shapes (circle, star) in the four corners, with matching colors or shapes on the display. The approach may also be extended by dividing the interface frame into eight areas.

Developing a Hand Pointing Response. Hand pointing is often the first response method considered. It is a normally occurring act which may already be in the nonspeaker's repertoire and has a high probability of acceptance by nonspeakers and their communication partners. However, for many nonspeakers, hand pointing will be inefficient. Table 11.3 presents several factors to be considered in assessing hand pointing ability and provides sample modifications for improving its efficiency.

Selecting the Initial Lexicon

First graders have vocabulary sizes ranging from 2,500 to 26,000 words depending on the research methodology used (Lorge & Chall, 1963). Clearly even the lowest figure, 2500, is far too many entries for a communication display. Thus, unless the nonspeaker uses a symbolic language code such as the alphabet, the lexicon selection may involve some highly limit-

TABLE 11.3
Optimizing a Hand Pointing Response

FACTORS	SAMPLE CONSIDERATIONS	SAMPLE ADAPTATIONS

RANGE	Size of effective area
	Movement patterns
	Effect on opposite extremity
		Alter height and angle of
		  display
		Place entries in optimal
		  positions
		Alter size of display

ACCURACY	Ability to isolate
	  thumb/fingers
	Potential item spacing
	Visual monitoring of hand
		Use weight cuff
		Use appliance (e.g., T-stick)
		Place guard on display
		Alter size/spacing of entries
		Encourage middle finger
		  pointing

SPEED	Length of response time
	Area for quickest response
		Use sliding pointer, to main-
		  tain hand on board
		Alter organization of entries
		Place frequent entries in
		  quickly reached positions

EFFORT	Reasonableness of effort
	Motivation of user
	Overflow movements
		Use stability bar for nonpoint-
		  ing hand
		Use sliding pointer, to keep
		  hand in pointing position
		Reassess positioning (e.g., use
		  of strap for head control)

Adapted from Jewell and McDowell-Fleming (1984) and Musselwhite and St. Louis (1982).

ing choices, and each item selected must undergo rigorous examination. In some cases, selection of a system (e.g., PIC) will severely limit the potential pool, due to the small corpus of the symbol set. Table 11.4 synthesizes a variety of lexical selection strategies. Instructions for use must accompany all visual displays, as well as a means for indicating missing entries (e.g., a blank card). The chapter by Blau (1983) is especially instructive for readers desiring further discussion of both general and specific strategies.

Organizing the Display

Even the most functional lexical items may not be effectively and efficiently used if the display is poorly organized. This section will focus on yielding the optimal display of entries so that users may communicate as accurately, specifically, and rapidly as possible.

TABLE 11.4
Strategies for Selecting Initial Lexicons

STRATEGY	RATIONALE	EXAMPLE
Develop a Basic Word Pool	Ensures wide range for consideration	Training manuals Core lexicon
Conduct an Environmental Inventory		
Frequency of occurrence across people/places/ things/times	Opportunities for practice and generalization	CHAIR + GO + HAT −
High interest/dislike value	Allows environmental control	MUSIC + BATH −
User-selected items	For users with metalin- guistic skills	MAMA PLEASE WAIT
Bodily needs/feelings	Must be fulfilled before other communication	HURT YUCK HAPPY RATS
Examine Symbol Sets		
Transparency/iconicity of items	Enhances acquisition and interpretation	Amer-Ind: CRY + PIC: OLD −
Ease of production (for gestures)	Clear ones likely recog- nized, reinforced	Gestures in reper- toire are easier BRUSH +
Perceptual complexity	Numerous details may confuse users/partners	ASL: EAT + Picsyms: THEIR −
Asess Item Functionality		
Coding variety of functions	One word for com- ment/request	DRINK
Potential multiword combos	Rapid growth of output	MORE + BOUNCE −
Promotes peer interaction	Enhance social skills	jokes + TOILET −

Adapted from: Blau, 1983; Carlson, 1981a; Fristoe and Lloyd; Lahey and Bloom, 1977; Musselwhite and St. Louis, 1982.

Type of Display.   Nonelectronic displays can take on a variety of forms. The *single sheet display*, perhaps the most familiar, permits all entries to be visible, reducing demands on memory and physical manipulation (e.g., turning cards), often at the expense of a reduced number of entries. *Multiple displays* can involve flipping entire sheets to present additional entries, such as a set of single sheet displays, or arranging entries in columns and flipping columns (e.g., verbs) as needed. *Combination dis-*

plays present, for example, a single sheet with highly used entries, plus a flip card section for less frequent entries. Another option is for the user to indicate a category, such as people, after which the user or communication partner turns to the appropriate page in a *supplemental notebook*, offering an array of further entries for providing more specific information.

The use of topical *miniboards* (e.g., array of fast food entries) or duplicate displays can allow for extended vocabulary appropriate to a variety of situations and settings. Table 11.5 presents several communication displays that might stimulate further ideas.

Format of Display. This concerns the physical arrangement of entries on the display, and strategies for improving access to them. For example, if the alphabet is to be used, an alphabetic, typewriter, or other arrangement must be selected. Beukelman and Yorkston (1982) found that arranging letters in the upper left area of the display according to frequency of occurrence results in a communication rate that is 26% faster than an A–Z arrangement. The Fitzgerald Key, developed to teach sentence structure to deaf children, is often used in displays. Entries are placed in columns

TABLE 11.5
Samples of Innovative Communication Displays

DESCRIPTION OF DISPLAY	SAMPLE ENTRIES	SETTING/SITUATION
Fishing tackle box	2″ × 2″ objects	Training; play
Apron or T-shirt (for user/partner)	P.T. vocabulary Arts & crafts entries	Physical therapy Art
Gallon milk jug with top cut out for scooping	Bath symbols Sand play symbols	Tub or pool Sandbox or beach
Placemat	Eating & activity words	Mealtime
Toy play board	Farm animals, actions Locations (COW/GO/IN)	Toy barn set Zoo set
Song strips	Key words from songs	Music/circle time
Meal tray "twin"	Drawing of actual tray	Mealtime
Slide album pages	TV programs, comments (FUNNY, YUCK, WOW, LOOK)	Near television Video game time

Adapted from Carlson (1981b) and Musselwhite (1984).

by grammatical form (e.g., who, action, little word, added word, what, where, when) to promote rapid production of grammatical sentences.

Placement of entries on the display can enhance or impair access, especially for nonspeakers using direct selection. McDonald (1980b) cautions against the natural tendency to arrange the symbols in neat rows on a rectangular tray because this arrangement is not appropriate for all nonspeakers. Areas easily accessed may be prime locations for placement of highly used symbols, while some tray areas should not include any entries. The size, spacing, and boldness of entries must also be determined, based on assessment of the nonspeaker's motoric ability, visual skills, and the type of symbols to be used. McDonald (1980a) and Myers, Grows, Coleman, & Cook (1980) describe a number of assessment techniques to assist in making decisions concerning the format.

As with the content, certain organizational "tricks" may increase the available number of entries. For example, once the size of the square has been determined, two entries may be placed in that square, with the more frequently-used one colored black and the other red. Directions affixed to the display instruct the partner that, unless otherwise indicated, the user is pointing to the black entry. Thus, the number of entries per unit space can be doubled.

Introducing Conventional Symbol Use

Several general strategies should be considered when initiating symbol training. *Naturally-structured techniques*, focusing on events that are, or at least appear to be, naturally-occurring, should be emphasized over *artificially-structured techniques*, which use rote instruction apart from context (Musselwhite & St. Louis, 1982). This will encourage the use of interactive, communication-based techniques from the outset, and will help nonspeakers observe the power of communication. Emphasize expressive use of a symbol from the beginning, rather than requiring long periods of symbol comprehension training before the power of that symbol can be experienced. Use natural consequences instead of artificial reinforcement whenever possible. For example, "You showed me baby. Here she is. Can she kiss you?" would be a more appropriate and enjoyable response than "Good pointing. You found the baby."

Using Objects to Introduce Symbols. Although a mental age of 18 months is generally suggested as the minimum age for introducing conventional graphic symbols (Shane, 1981), preliminaries to symbol use may be initiated earlier. For example, younger children may be taught to select desired items or events by choosing appropriate objects. As Bottorf and DePape (1982) note, the partner's inconsistent presentations and responses to the child's selections are crucial. For example, a "5-bite-rule" for providing choices during mealtime has proven highly effective because aides find it reasonable to offer visual choices between food items or food and drink for the first five bites, with choices verified and responded to immediately ("You looked at the juice. Here it is."). Other choice situations are: play time (which toy?); dressing (which skirt?); and therapy (which activity first?).

Various authors have suggested specific strategies for moving from objects to graphic representations. Several exemplary strategies are summarized below:

1. *Use snack cartons* to represent snacks, starting with the 3-D carton, then reducing it to two dimensions (Shane, 1981).
2. *Take an instant photograph*, allowing the nonspeaker to watch it develop; point back and forth from symbol to referent (McDonald, 1980b).
3. *Trace around an object* (e.g., small doll) while the child watches; point back and forth from symbol to referent.
4. *Set up a training hierarchy* (e.g., Montgomery, 1980; Van Tatenhove, 1979); for example, when the nonspeaker indicates an object, he or she should receive the following, at successive steps; exact item indicated; exact replica of item indicated; nonidentical match (e.g., larger or different-colored ball); event indicated (e.g., chance to play ball). Object to photo/picture/symbol matches can then be initiated.

Enhancing Symbol Identification. Modification of the symbols and the environment can also aid in symbol acquisition. Below are sample strategies for assisting in symbol identification:

1. *Accentuate symbol iconicity* by adding details and/or colors; for example, the Picsym for HAND can be simply drawn with lines representing fingers, or details indicating flesh, knuckles, and fingernails can be added.
2. *Label the environment* (Bottorf & DePape, 1982), requesting partners to model use of symbols when appropriate.
3. *Increase the intensity* of a target symbol relative to decoys, or of key symbol elements relative to the background. The Picsyms pronouns depict the key figure in solid lines, while the background figures are drawn with dotted or lightened lines (see symbol for HER in Figure 11.2). This tactic can be applied to other systems, fading the intensity when possible.

Enhancing Communicative Interactions. Parents and the professional staff who work with nonspeaking children are aware that communication displays are not used as frequently or as effectively as had been hoped. Yoder and Kraat (1983) concluded after a review of the few available studies of interaction between other persons and users of communication displays that nonspeakers have fewer opportunities to communicate, communicate less frequently, and are given but one utterance per turn.

Barriers to Effective Interaction

Aided communication systems may impose barriers to effective communication. Sample barriers noted (Harris, 1982; Yoder and Kraat, 1983) include:

1. *The communication techniques and symbols selected:* Techniques may interfere with eye contact, and symbols may be difficult to interpret.
2. *Altered conversational patterns:* Speaker/listener roles and turn-taking protocols may be drastically changed if the listener participates in message formulation, giving a great power advantage to the listener.
3. *Altered temporal patterns:* "Real conversational time," or production of a message at the rate of oral communication, is necessary for aspects of conversation such as commenting on fast-moving action; this may be impossible with many aided systems. A slow rate may also result in loss of listener attention, shift of topic, or listener interruption.
4. *Altered conversational forms and functions:* The need for brevity may force nonspeakers to abandon polite forms and humor to allow rapid message transmission; communication partners may produce a preponderance of requests and directives, with less use of conversational functions such as information sharing and commenting.

Strategies for Enhancing Interaction

Bottorf and DePape (1982) stress that "Ignoring previously effective modes of expression may have a negative effect on both the nonspeaking person's and others' acceptance of the new system" (p. 58). Therefore, they recommend several approaches for assessing interaction and modifying existing styles. This section will focus on general and specific strategies for enhancing interaction, with the caution that existing strategies should be incorporated if appropriate.

General Strategies.   The emphasis on naturally-structured rather than artificially-structured techniques (Musselwhite & St. Louis, 1982) was discussed earlier in this chapter. This approach involves reduced use of drills in favor of more naturalistic activities, and suggests modifications of necessary drills to make them more communicative. For example, "show speech," or speech that is for display rather than communication, can be minimized by asking the nonspeaker to practice formulating comments (IT'S RED) or exchanging information (YOU RIDE ON IT) about pictures unseen by the communication partner. While still a drill-type activity, the pair is involved in true communication, and the partner has the added task of decoding an unknown message.

Constable (1983) provides a number of excellent general strategies for creating communicative context through techniques such as:

1. *Creating nonlinguistic support:* The facilitator should draw attention to the environment by gesturing to referents, then removing objects to encourage requesting.
2. *Using environmental engineering or "creative stupidity":* This technique involves setting up situations so that the nonspeaker has a need or a desire to communicate. Samples are: violating routine events (e.g., trying to paint with waterless powder); withholding objects like paintbrushes or turns to pleasant activities such as tickling; violating object function or manipulation (e.g., pushing a car on its top). In these examples, the nonspeaker would have a purpose for requesting objects (NEED, WATER), requesting events (TICKLE PLEASE), or commenting on actions (UH-OH, CAR ON TOP).

Closely related to these strategies is the general tactic of *building shared scripts* around routine events such as mealtime, to encourage discussion of familiar topics. Through shared scripts, adults or peer models can put vocabulary (MORE), structure (MORE _____), or communicative functions (informing: TIME TO EAT) on display. Once the nonspeaker has learned the basic script, the communication partner can encourage him or her to participate by setting up a situation, then delaying and looking expectant. The facilitator should also *introduce new events*, such as pet therapy, to serve as new topics. The emphasis placed on these two approaches to topic introduction depends on the maturity, interests, and needs of the nonspeaker. The major focus of all these general interaction strategies is to encourage the nonspeaker to initiate communication and to be a more equal communication partner, even during training.

Specific Strategies. Some interaction needs or problems of nonspeakers may require more specific techniques. Strategies for meeting several identified needs are summarized below.

Maximizing Communicative Modes. It is commonly accepted that no single device can replace the richness of communication through speech. Therefore, nonspeakers should be trained to use supplementary modes that are unambiguous, add to the message, and are not distracting. For example, pointing, head-shaking, and vocalizing agreement are all normative supplemental modes used by speakers. Table 11.6 presents a summary of four communication modes and a sampling of nonspeech strategies to optimize use of each mode.

TABLE 11.6
Strategies for Maximizing Use of Four Communication Modes

MODE	DESCRIPTION	NONSPEECH STRATEGIES FOR TURN HOLDING[a]
LANGUAGE	Includes phonemic, syntactic, and semantic categories	Point to LET ME FINISH on communication display
PARALINGUISTICS	Vocal aspects of communication (e.g., articulation control, stress, intonation)	Possibly loud vocalization to inhibit listener Likely difficult for nonspeakers
KINESICS	Bodily movements and postures occurring during communication	"Stop" gestures; reaching for listener's arm
PROXEMICS	Interpersonal distance	Invading listener's space to maintain turn (Not possible for many nonspeakers)

Adapted from Higginbotham and Yoder (1982)
[a]Higginbotham and Yoder (1982) include verbal and nonverbal components for a variety of turn rules and functions (e.g., turn claiming/yielding).

Preventing/Repairing Communication Breakdowns. Blau (1983) asserts that "A frequent source of communication breakdown between speaking and nonspeaking people is the speaker's underestimation of the nonspeaker's cognitive status" (p. 230). She suggests that this may result from lack of "back-channel" responses (similar to "Oh, I see"), signaled by the nonspeaker to indicate that the message is being received. These may be linguistic (TELL ME MORE), paralinguistic (approximation of UH-HUH), or kinesic (smile, head nod). Similarly, the partner must provide back-channel responses to the nonspeaker, perhaps by verbalizing the message as it is indicated. Bottorf and DePape (1982) recommend that the system user should decide issues such as the preferred listener feedback and signals to indicate misunderstanding. This information can then be included in the instructions block on the display.

Role playing is a general strategy recommended for preventing or repairing communication breakdowns. Nonspeakers can thus learn what to expect from unfamiliar partners (e.g., frequent wrong guesses), and how to prevent these difficulties (e.g., point to instructions PLEASE DON'T

GUESS), or reestablish communication (e.g., repeating, using initial cueing, or another mode).

Training Communication Partners.   Even minimal training of potential partners may yield great success in enhancing interaction. For example, Calculator and Luchko (1983) found that a one-half hour inservice to nursing home staff and residents contributed greatly to increasing interaction for an adult nonspeaker with normal intelligence. The brief inservice stressed: close proximity, demonstrating to the nonspeaker that his or her board was useful (e.g., by complying with her requests), using open-ended *wh*-questions, and evaluating the content and context when she did not respond. Other areas to cover in training partners are:

1. Common communication errors to avoid such as: Using "baby talk"; altering pitch range, loudness level, or rate; asking questions to which answers are self-evident; and conversing only on superficial topics such as school or weather (Montgomery, 1980).
2. Use of feedback and message completion techniques (e.g., finishing the message as soon as the nonspeaker's intent becomes clear) appropriate for and acceptable to the nonspeaker.
3. Strategies to assist in repairing breakdowns (i.e., when failure to understand the nonspeaker's message occurs), such as requesting a repeat or a message reformulation ("Could you spell it?").

Enhancing Peer Interaction.   In a study of communicative interaction with nonspeaking severely physically disabled children, Harris (1982) found that children rarely interacted with peers. Several tactics designed to increase interaction with both nonspeaking and speaking peers are:

1. Provide mini-boards for conversing about play activities. Each mini-board would be self-contained, and would include less than 30 message items. The following examples illustrate sample words and phrases appropriate for the specific play situations: sandbox (POUR, BUCKET); video games (MY TURN, GOTCHA!); card games (GIVE ME ALL YOUR _____; RATS!).
2. Inform one partner that the other has a secret message to share ("Janie's going somewhere really special!").
3. Help nonspeakers role play methods to resolve breakdowns when neither has access to vocal output.

REFERENCES

ASHA Ad Hoc Committee on Communication Processes and Nonspeaking Persons. (1981). Position statement on nonspeech communication. *ASHA, 23,* 577–581.
Baker, B. (1983). Chopsticks and Beethoven. *Communication Outlook, 5,* 8–10.

Beukelman, D. R., & Yorkston, K. M. (1977). A communication system for the severely dysarthric speaker with an intact language system. *Journal of Speech and Hearing Disorders, 41*, 265–270.

Beukelman, D. R., & Yorkston, K. M. (1982). Communication interaction of adult communication augmentation system use. *Topics in Language Disorders, 2*, 39–53.

Blau, A. (1983). Vocabulary selection in augmentative communication: Where do we begin? In H. Winitz (Ed.), *Treating language disorders: For clinicians by clinicians* (pp. 205–232). Austin, TX: PRO-ED.

Bottorf, L., & DePape, D. (1982). Initiating communication systems for severely speech-impaired persons. *Topics in Language Disorders, 2*, 55–71.

Calculator, S., & Luchko, C. (1983). Evaluating the effectiveness of a communication board training program. *Journal of Speech and Hearing Disorders, 48*, 185–191.

Carlson, F. (1981a). A format for selecting vocabulary for the nonspeaking child. *Language Speech Hearing Services in Schools, 12*, 240–245.

Carlson, F. (1981b). *Alternate methods of communication: A handbook for students and clinicians.* Danville, IL: The Interstate Printers and Publishers.

Clark, C. R., Davies, C. O., & Woodcock, R. W. (1974). *Standard rebus glossary.* Circle Pines, MN: American Guidance Service.

Clark, R. (1984). *Verbal eyes verbalize.* Unpublished manuscript.

Constable, C. (1983). Creating communicative context. In H. Winitz (Ed.), *Treating language disorders: For clinicians by clinicians* (pp. 97–120). Austin, TX: PRO-ED.

Daniloff, J. K., Lloyd, L. L., & Fristoe, M. (1983). Amer-Ind transparency. *Journal of Speech and Hearing Disorders, 48*, 103–110.

Duffy, L. (1977). *An innovative approach to the development of communication skills for severely speech handicapped cerebral palsied children.* Unpublished master's thesis, University of Nevada, Las Vegas.

Fristoe, M., & Lloyd, L. L. (1980). Planning an initial expressive sign lexicon for persons with severe communication impairment. *Journal of Speech and Hearing Disorders, 45*, 170–180.

Goodenough-Trepagnier, C., & Prather, P. (1979). *Manual for teachers of SPEEC.* Boston: Tufts-New England Medical Center.

Goodenough-Trepagnier, C., & Prather, P. (1981). Communication systems for the nonvocal based on frequent phoneme sequences. *Journal of Speech Hearing Research, 45*, 170–180.

Goodenough-Trepagnier, C., Tarry, E., & Prather, P. (1982). Derivation of an efficient nonvocal communication system. *Human Factors, 24*, 163–172.

Harris, D. (1982). Communicative interaction processes involving nonvocal physically handicapped children. *Topics in Language Disorders, 2*, 21–37.

Harris, D., & Vanderheiden, G. (1980). Enhancing the development of communication interaction. In R. Schiefelbush (Ed.), *Nonspeech language and communication: Analysis and intervention* (pp. 227–257). Austin, TX: PRO-ED.

Hehner, B. (1980). *Blissymbols for use.* Toronto, Canada: Blissymbolics Communication Institute.

Henegar, M. G., & Cornett, R. O. (1981). *Cued speech handbook for parents.* Washington, DC: Cued Speech Program, Gallaudet College.

Higginbotham, D. J., & Yoder, C. E. (1982). Communication within natural conversational interaction: Implications for severe communicatively impaired persons. *Topics in Language Disorders, 2*, 1–19.

Hoemann, H. W. (1975). The transparency of meaning of sign language gestures. *Sign Language Studies, 7*, 151–161.

Jewell, K., & McDowell-Fleming, M. (1984). *Evaluation of hand skills of non-verbal athetoid CP children: Treatment implications.* Paper presented at the meeting of the North Carolina Augmentative Communication Association, Lenox Baker Children's Hospital, Durham, NC.

Jones, L. V., & Wepman, J. M. (1966). *A spoken word count.* Chicago: Language Research Associates.

Kiernan, C., Reid, B., & Jones, L. (1979). Signs and symbols: Who uses what? *Special Education: Forward Trends, 6,* 32–34.

Kollinzas, G. (1983). The communication record: Sharing information to promote sign language generalization. *Journal of the Association for Severely Handicapped, 8,* 49–55.

Lahey, M., & Bloom, L. (1977). Planning a first lexicon: Which words to teach first. *Journal of Speech and Hearing Disorders, 42,* 340–350.

Lloyd, L. (1982). Symbol and initial lexica selection. *Proceedings of the Second International Conference on Non-Speech Communication,* 9–15. Toronto: Ontario Institute for Studies in Education.

Lorge, I., and Chall, J. (1963). Estimating the size of vocabularies of children and adults: An analysis of methodological issues. *Journal of Experimental Education, 32,* 147–157.

McDonald, E. T. (1980a). *Teaching and using Blissymbolics.* Toronto, Canada: The Blissymbolics Communication Institute.

McDonald, E. T. (1980b). Early identification and treatment of children at risk for speech development. In R. L. Schiefelbusch (Ed.), *Nonspeech language and communication: Analysis and intervention* (pp. 49–79). Austin, TX: PRO-ED.

McNaughton, S., & Kates, B.. (1980). The application of Blissymbolics. In R. L. Schiefelbusch (Ed.), *Nonspeech language and communication: Analysis and intervention* (pp. 303–321). Baltimore: University Park Press.

Montgomery, J. (Ed.). (1980). *Non-oral communication: A training guide for the child without speech.* Fountain Valley, CA: Fountain Valley School District.

Musselwhite, C. (1982). *A comparison of three symbolic communication systems.* Unpublished doctoral dissertation, West Virginia University.

Musselwhite, C. (1986). *Adaptive play for special needs children: Strategies to embrace communication and learning.* Austin, TX: PRO-ED.

Musselwhite, C., & Ruscello, D. (1984). The transparency of three communication symbol systems. *Journal of Speech Hearing Research, 27,* 436–443.

Musselwhite, C., & St. Louis, K. W. (1982). *Communication programming for the severely handicapped: Vocal and non-vocal strategies.* San Diego, CA: College-Hill Press.

Myers, L. S., Grows, N. L., Coleman, C. L., & Cook, A. M. (1980). *An assessment battery for assistive device systems recommendations, Part 1.* Sacramento, CA: California State University, Assistive Device Center.

Shane, H. (1981). Decision making in early augmentative communication system use. In R. Schiefelbusch & D. Bricker (Eds.), *Early Language: Acquisition and intervention* (pp. 389–425). Austin, TX: PRO-ED.

Shane, H., & Bashir, A. (1980). Election criteria for determining candidacy for an augmentative communication system: Preliminary considerations. *Journal of Speech and Hearing Disorders, 45,* 408–414.

Silverman, F. (1980). *Communication for the speechless.* Englewood Cliffs, NJ: Prentice-Hall.

Silverman, H., McNaughton, S., and Kates, B. (1978). *Handbook of Blissymbolics for Instructors, Users, Parents and Administrators.* Toronto, Canada: Blissymbolics Communication Institute.

Skelly, M. (1979). *Amer-Ind gestural code based on universal American Indian hand talk*. New York: Elsevier-North Holland.

Van Tatenhove, G. (1979). *Augmentative communication system development: A response training protocol*. Paper presented at the American Speech-Language-Hearing Association Convention, Atlanta, GA.

Warrick, A. (1982). Look at me—I'm talking to you: A discussion on eye pointing. *Proceedings of the Second International Conference on Non-Speech Communication*, 78–80. Toronto: Ontario Institute for Studies in Education.

Yoder, D., & Kraat, A. (1983). Intervention issues in nonspeech communication. In J. Miller, D. Yoder, & R. Schiefelbusch (Eds.), *Contemporary issues in language intervention* (pp. 27–51). Rockville, MD: American Speech-Language-Hearing Association.

CHAPTER 12

Educational Programming

Lura G. Parker

Many aspects of development are adversely affected by cerebral palsy, and because children are affected in different ways, each child is unique. Individualized educational programs must be developed, curriculum planning must take into consideration the special needs of cerebral palsied children, and teaching methods must be tailored to the needs and abilities of each child.

1. *What are the provisions of the* Education for All Handicapped Children Act *(PL 94–142), and how do they affect educational programming for children with cerebral palsy?*

2. *What are the advantages and disadvantages of each of the educational settings described by Parker? Why might the "least restrictive" setting not be the best educational placement for a cerebral palsied child?*

3. *Why might grouping be important in the educational program for a cerebral palsied child, and what methods of grouping might be used in the classroom?*

4. *In addition to the child's cognitive level and motor problems, what other factors does Parker suggest be considered when planning the educational program?*

INTRODUCTION

Today all cerebral palsied children, regardless of the severity of their neuromuscular dysfunction or the nature of their associated problems, are entitled to a free and appropriate education. The term *education* has come to mean not only the three R's—reading, 'riting, and 'rithmetic—but any training that can be given a handicapped child to meet his or her individual needs. Thus, for one child an appropriate education may include learning the basic skills of dressing, toileting, and communication; for another it may include learning to walk with crutches as well as learning the more traditional academic subjects.

Yet providing appropriate educational experiences for the cerebral palsied has proven a complex and demanding task. Cerebral palsy is one of the most complicated disabilities known. It not only affects motor performance but also may involve hearing, sight, speech, seizure activity, and intellectual functioning. As with the motor patterns, the degree of involvement ranges from minimal to severe. There is no typical person with cerebral palsy. The more one deals with cerebral palsy, the more aware he is of the individual reactions to the limitations imposed. Because of this wide diversification, no educational program or practice is universally appropriate. Just as each person with cerebral palsy is unique, each educational program must be unique—individualized—to meet the appropriate needs.

It is the uniqueness that dictates the range of program options needed to serve the cerebral palsied adequately. Yet even within this range, significant individualization must occur.

EDUCATION FOR ALL HANDICAPPED CHILDREN ACT (PL 94-142)

Until recent years educational opportunities for children with cerebral palsy were limited. In many localities very young handicapped children and children possessing severe handicaps could not obtain services. In addition, the quality of existing services varied greatly from place to place. In some instances the needs of each individual child were pinpointed and the teachers and therapists addressed those needs. In other instances, little appropriate instruction occurred.

The Mandate

In November, 1975, the Education of All Handicapped Children Act, Public Law (PL) 94-142, was enacted guaranteeing the right of every child—regardless of handicapping condition—to a free and appropriate education. The law mandated that appropriate educational programs be made available to each child and ensured program quality by requiring an individualized education plan (IEP). A portion of the law specified safeguards to protect the rights of children and parents. In several of these safeguards the teacher plays an important role. These safeguards include:

A Free Appropriate Public Education. The law makes educational opportunities available to all exceptional children between the ages of 3 and 21. The assurance of an appropriate education guarantees that the child, whether pursuing an academic course or developing self-help skills, will be included in the educational system and instructed appropriately. "Child Find," a systematic search to identify children in need of specialized services, is also a part of this safeguard. In most communities "Child Find" concentrates on screening the preschool population for possible identification and referral.

The Right to Due Process. Included is a series of steps which assures the right of the parents and child to be fully informed and to participate in decision making, evaluation, placement, instruction, and re-evaluation. These procedures apply in any and all decisions concerning the handicapped child's schooling and require prior consultation with the child's parents or guardian.

Nondiscriminatory Testing. Included is the assurance that special placement is to be decided on the basis of evaluation, materials, and procedures appropriate for such purposes and that no single test or procedure is to be used as the sole criterion for placement. The test and other evaluation materials used in placing exceptional children are to be administered in such a way as not to be racially or culturally discriminatory and must be presented in the native language of the child.

Least Restrictive Environment. The law provides the assurance that exceptional children are to be educated with nonexceptional children to the maximum extent appropriate. Exceptional children are to be placed in separate or special classes or schools only when the nature or severity of the exceptionality is such that education in regular classes cannot be achieved satisfactorily.

Confidentiality. The law provides that any information contained in school records will not be released without the permission of the parents.

Individualized Educational Program. The IEP is a written statement developed by school officials, teachers, parents or guardian, and the child. It includes the child's present achievement level, the long- and short-range annual goals, the extent of participation in regular programs, a timeline of the service provisions, a plan or schedule for checking the progress of the child, and consideration of needs for revision. The IEP is reviewed yearly.

Under PL 94-142 the most important area of focus for teachers is the implementation of IEP, for it is through this written statement that both the teacher and the parents establish goals and priorities for the child, thus creating an educational Master Plan for the year. While the IEP is one facet of the law, all six safeguards are interdependent and must be considered in the process of developing and implementing IEPs.

Effect of IEP on Educational Programming

It has been pointed out that the IEP is required by law. However, the primary reason for developing and implementing an IEP should not be merely to satisfy legal requirements. The IEP has strong educational value and can help improve educational practices. Some of the potential positive outcomes of the IEP development and implementation include the following areas.

Sequential Curriculum Development. In the past, teachers of handicapped students have been unsure which skills and concepts were appropriate to their students' needs when adaptations to the curriculum were necessary. As a result, handicapped students have often worked on lessons representing disjointed or random skill development. When the child had a change of teachers, the new teacher frequently had little idea of what skills the student had already mastered and, at times, there was needless teaching of skills which the child had already learned.

The IEP provides an opportunity for educators and parents to plan the child's program systematically. Adaptation to the curriculum and the appropriate sequential development of skills can be specified on the IEP. Future teachers can refer to old IEPs to note past goals and progress.

Coordination of Programming. The IEP is not developed by the teacher alone, but by a committee which includes the child's teacher, the parents, a school representative responsible for providing or supervising special education, and other persons requested by the parents or school. During planning, the committee has the opportunity to coordinate their efforts to ensure effective implementation. For example, if during the committee meeting, it is agreed that a child needs speech therapy, one committee member is made responsible for ensuring the child receives immediate service from a speech therapist. The IEP development also provides the opportunity for parent and teacher to coordinate their efforts.

Increased Attention to the Individual Needs of Students. Development of an IEP forces those persons who will be working with the child to meet and analyze systematically what assistance the child needs and how this assistance can be provided. For example, a young hearing-impaired preschooler with cerebral palsy will need to have new concepts presented by demonstration as well as verbally. A severely multiply handicapped teenager may need to be placed in specially adapted equipment before he can attend to stimuli. The IEP provides opportunities to make individual adaptations based on the needs of the students.

Specifications of Needed Services. An IEP must specify an appropriate educational program. Often for an educational program to be *appropriate*, it must include related services for handicapped students. These related services as defined in PL 94-142 include transportation, speech pathology and audiology, psychological services, physical and occupational therapy, recreation, early identification and assessment of disabilities, counseling services, and medical services for diagnostic or evaluation purposes. It is often those related services that remove the barriers to school success and enable a student to profit from specially designed instruction.

Systematic Evaluation. In the IEP a statement outlining the child's present level of performance is required. This description of the child's present level of functioning provides a basis for planning appropriate educational objectives.

Both long-range (annual) goals and short-term (instructional) objectives are stated in the IEP. These goals and objectives are designed so that the teacher and others working with the child know exactly what to teach the child. In the instructional objective a criterion for the mastery of the skill is included. For example, "Mary Jane McKay will match four alphabet letters to their corresponding objects four out of five times." By specifying the degree of accuracy necessary for the successful mastery of the skill (four out of five times) the teacher has a method of evaluating Mary Jane's progress on a continuing basis. Thus the IEP provides a means of systematic ongoing evaluation of the child's progress.

Increased Professional Accountability. The IEP is a statement of intent on the part of all those who are involved in its development and implementation. While it is not legally binding, educators are clearly expected to make good faith efforts to assist the child in meeting the goals of the IEP. When all those who develop the IEP give their formal approval they are sanctioning the IEP as representing an appropriate education for the handicapped child. The IEP can prevent misunderstandings at a later date between parent and teacher or teacher and agency over the precise nature of the child's instruction.

EDUCATIONAL SETTINGS

Educational opportunities are made available to the general population from the ages of 5 or 6 to 18. Most states now offer programs for the handicapped from 2 to 3 years of age to 21. In devising educational programs for the cerebral palsied, it is necessary to consider not only the child's chronological age but other factors which affect learning such as intellectual functioning, motor impairment, associated secondary handicaps, and present needs. In addition, PL 94-142 requires the child be placed in the most appropriate, *least restrictive* setting. No longer can the severity of handicap automatically dictate placement (Miller & Switzky, 1978). Four major types of educational settings are present: residential centers, specialized day treatment centers, self-contained classrooms, and mainstreamed classrooms.

Residential Centers

Public residential centers have traditionally served the most severely handicapped children. While originally such centers provided little educational or therapeutic opportunities, since the passage of PL 94-142 in 1975, these centers have had to provide appropriate learning experiences for their residents. A nationwide emphasis on deinstitutionalization has resulted in a drop in the number of persons living in these centers. For the most severely physically and mentally impaired persons with cerebral palsy, this placement continues as an option—even though cognitive and physical gains noticeably lag in this type setting (Bush, 1980). For some families the relief from constant care of the cerebral palsied can be the deciding advantage.

Private residential centers which specialize in the education and treatment of children with cerebral palsy have the disadvantage of separating the child from family and nonhandicapped peers. However, for many cerebral palsied children, this disadvantage is offset by the benefit of being taught and treated by well trained teachers and therapists. By bringing together in one facility a number of cerebral palsied children, staff members can gain extensive experience in evaluation, education, treatment, and other activities which comprise a comprehensive program.

Specialized Day Treatment Facilities

Specialized schools offering day programs to the cerebral palsied are usually run by local community agencies. The public schools contract with the specialized school to provide an educational program. Often the schools offer parental support groups as well as educational and therapeutic programs for the child. These day schools usually draw from a number of small school systems which have just a few cerebral palsied children. In large metropolitan areas, the public school itself may operate the specialized school.

The specialized day school has several advantages. First, the staff is familiar with the numerous problems that a child with cerebral palsy may exhibit. Second, the traditional therapies (physical, occupational, and speech) are more readily available because of the large number of children requiring this help. Third, parents are able to interact with other parents whose children have similar problems. The disadvantages include possible long commutes to school each day for the child and little contact with normal peers.

Self-Contained Classrooms

The self-contained classroom enrolls only handicapped children and operates within a school building for nonhandicapped children. Usually the student/teacher ratio is low. This setting may offer limited exposure to peers in the normalized setting (that is, lunch, music, school celebrations). To take advantage of these social-emotional opportunities, handicapped children under age 12 should be housed in an elementary school and those over age 12 should be placed in a junior or senior high even if their curriculum is not comparable with their peers in this secondary setting.

This setting offers the advantage of being less isolated than the day facility. Commutes to school are usually shorter. However, physical, occupational, and speech therapies may be less available. Since the self-contained class is located within the regular school building, it is essential that all school personnel and students be educated as to how to interact appropriately with the handicapped children. Some schools allow peer tutors. The nonhandicapped children may elect during lunch or a specified free time to feed a child or teach a concept. Teachers of handicapped children often complain of a feeling of isolation in this setting. Parents may lack a support network unless a parent program is initiated.

Mainstreamed Classrooms

The mainstreamed setting is the most controversial. The child with cerebral palsy attends class with his nonhandicapped peers. Support help in the form of a resource teacher, an aide for personal care, or a physical therapist may or may not be present. Usually the classroom teacher has had little training in exceptionality. The benefits to the handicapped child have been emphasized. Academics in this setting are stronger. Proponents feel mainstreaming is a microcosm of real world experiences and thus better prepares the handicapped child to cope in the future (Forness, 1977; Newberger, 1978). Success in large measure depends on the comfort level of the classroom teacher, the availability of support staff, and the acceptance of the handicapped child by his peers. Adjustment is facilitated if the child with cerebral palsy possesses a competency to which peers can relate, otherwise the handicapped child may be babied or ostracized.

A few years ago, two children were mainstreamed into a small public school system in North Carolina. Both had cerebral palsy. Martha was ambulatory although markedly ataxic, verbal, and had learning disabilities. Jane was nonambulatory, had poor coordination of her upper extremities, and used a communication board to augment her barely understandable speech. Surprisingly, it was Jane who was readily accepted. Her ability in mathematics gave her a competency to which the other children could relate. She soon became the child the others gravitated toward for math answers. Jane was included in activities in the lunch room and on the playground. Martha, on the other hand, although more mildly handicapped, was ostracized. She *physically* and *mentally* was different from her peers thus giving her no competency. Her classmates did not consider her an "equal."

The advantages and disadvantages of mainstreaming are still being debated (Jones, Gottlieb, Guskin, & Yoshida, 1978). It appears to work extremely well for some and to be disastrous for others. The decision to mainstream a child should be made on an individual basis (Heron, 1978). The mainstreamed child enjoys the benefits of an academically oriented program, the companionship of neighborhood children, and a usually shorter commute. Therapeutic services are not as readily available and parent support groups are usually nonexistent.

In considering any educational setting, it is important to remember that no child should be locked into a particular placement. A variety of educational settings over the child's educational lifetime may be required. Continuing re-evaluation of the child's needs is necessary to ensure the appropriate placement.

EDUCATIONAL PRACTICES

Considerations in Developing Curriculum Materials

With normally developing children, the curriculum is supplied to the teachers and expectations and goals are recognized community-wide. Kindergartners should know their ABCs by year's end; third graders their multiplication tables; fifth graders the U.S. states and capitals. When teaching cerebral palsied children, it may be necessary to modify content, materials, and methods. A teacher cannot assume that because Johnny is 10 he is ready to write a book report. Indeed, Johnny may not even be able to hold a pencil! Because cerebral palsy affects each child differently, few generalizations can be made. Physically and mentally, children with cerebral palsy represent a wide range of abilities. It is helpful to consider certain factors when developing education materials for the cerebral palsied.

Isolation From Normal Experience. Because of their physical limitations, cerebral palsied children may not have interacted with toys or the environment in the same way or to the same extent as their peers. The puzzles and tricycles of the preschool years and video games of the elementary years may be too difficult motorically or cognitively. Lack of opportunities to manipulate items in the environment, to learn from cause/effect relationships, and to refine perceptual skills impacts adversely on learning.

To reduce the isolation imposed by the handicap, toys and games must be adapted and specially structured play and recreation opportunities provided. For preschoolers, several children positioned around a sand or water table may be effective. If necessary, assist the child in the manipulation of cups, funnels, etc. Suspend a soft ball from the ceiling. Children can hit it with their arms or legs, and the ball will return without the child's having to fetch it. Older children can play board games or cards. If necessary, have a "helper" assist the cerebral palsied children move the marker or card allowing the handicapped child to make all the decisions regarding the play of the game. These decisions can help recreationally reinforce academic concepts. Computers also offer an avenue for recreational as well as academic learning. Many programs are available that allow the cerebral palsied child with only one controllable motion to mix or match shapes, play checkers, or logic games.

Social or Group Interactions.   Many children with cerebral palsy have not had group experiences. Socially the child may be immature, unable to wait his turn or communicate effectively in a group setting. The classroom should be a place where an effort is made not only to individualize work but to incorporate the child into group activities. It is necessary for the cerebral palsied child to develop socially and as a member of the group. So many times, the school experience is the only group experience the child has.

There are various ways to group children. Different types of groups are appropriate for the teaching of different things. The following is a description of several ways of grouping that might be included in the classroom:

Grouping by Skill.   The children are grouped according to skills they are working on (e.g., fine motor, cognitive, language, writing, or gross motor). In some classrooms specific areas are designated for certain skills.

Grouping by Behaviors.   The children are grouped on the basis of their appropriate or inappropriate behaviors. For example, John who is very aggressive and does not like to sit in a chair is grouped with Denise who has good attending skills and likes to do her small group work. Denise will serve as a model for John.

Grouping All Together.   The children are given an opportunity to relate to each other and their teachers in a structured situation. They are taught to "wait" and "speak" in front of a group, to "listen to others speak," and other social skills.

Grouping by Activity.   The children are given an opportunity to choose one activity from among a group of two more activities. This type of grouping is informal and nonstructured in terms of direct teaching. "Free play" times throughout a day are often done this way.

Static Environment. A handicapped child's environment is often more static than that of a normally developing child. Outings should be planned to acquaint the child with the community.

Pictures in the classroom should be rotated frequently. For nonambulatory children, the same wall may be a constant focal point. Ensure that the child has something worthwhile to view. If the child is positioned in a travel or recliner chair, check to see the level of the eye gaze. It may differ from the ambulatory child's. For those children positioned frequently on the floor or a mat, place and rotate items at their eye level.

Self-Image. Many children with cerebral palsy do not possess positive self-images. They have tried and failed repeatedly at tasks. Others' reactions to them are internalized, family members may view them not as a contributing member of the constellation, but as an object of continual care. Strangers may react in a negative manner by ignoring or infantilizing them.

A poor self-image interferes with optimal learning efficiency. Symptoms that the child may exhibit include: general unhappiness with no specific cause, unwillingness to attempt new tasks or repeat tasks that were failed previously, withdrawal, and aggressive behavior.

To facilitate the construction of a more positive outlook, the teacher should structure specific opportunities where the child can succeed—by asking in the group setting a question to which the child knows the answer, giving worksheets that contain some material that the child has already mastered, praising the child's accomplishments to others, etc.

The teacher needs to give clear signals as to her expectations of the child. When the handicapped child realizes someone else believes he can do it, that instills confidence. Encouragement should be given to the child to assume certain responsibilities or jobs which, in turn, are a reinforcement of the child's importance to the functioning of the classroom—an ambulatory child might erase the board while a severely handicapped child might throw away unwanted papers by pushing them off his lap board and allowing them to fall in a large trash box.

A positive self-image helps the handicapped child develop effective relationships with others. The child can then exert more energy and enthusiasm into the process of learning and growing as an individual.

Factors Affecting Teaching Methods

A significant number of children with cerebral palsy have identified learning problems such as distractibility, perseveration, and perceptual difficulties. While not unique to the cerebral palsy population, learning problems make implementing an appropriate educational program even more complicated. In addition, fatigue and speech distortions add to the list affecting teaching methods.

Distractibility. Distractibility, or the inability of the child to focus attention on the task at hand, is a major learning problem for many cerebral palsied children (Vance, 1980). This characteristic may be referred to as hyperactivity or excitability. Whatever the label, the problem is serious as it interferes with the child's ability to concentrate and absorb information efficiently. A quiet corner is essential. As many extraneous stimulants as possible should be screened out. The child requires assistance in attending and concentrating. A behavior-shaping program where the rewards are frequent and consequences of failing to stay on task are consistent appears to be the most effective means of controlling this problem.

Perseveration. Perseveration, sometimes regarded as the opposite of distractibility, is characterized by difficulty shifting attention from one task or set to another. This sometimes is mistaken for stubbornness. When a child appears to be perseverating, it is helpful to give cues. Verbally remind the child before task completion as to what he should do next. "Johnny, when you reach the end of the page, close your book and look at me." Give a specific ending point. Avoid allowing him to work too much on his own thus creating opportunities for the behavior to continue. Again, as in distractibility, rewards for the appropriate behaviors are important as well as consistency in dealing with the inappropriate actions. Class time routines often help as well as auditory signals such as the ringing of the bell. (See Smith (1983) for additional information.)

Speech. Some cerebral palsied children, particularly those with athetosis, may have hard-to-understand speech, limited speech, or no intelligible vocalizations. Difficulty in communicating effectively and efficiently can cause undesirable behaviors in the affected child. At times the child may cry easily from frustration or as a means of securing attention. Many of these children withdraw or are less willing to participate in activities requiring communication, particularly those in group settings. The teacher should be aware of these responses and structure activities that raise the communication comfort level for the child. For the child with limited or garbled speech, the teacher might ask questions requiring only one word or a short answer. As the child feels more at ease in being able to relate his thoughts, the teacher can extend his or her expectations. However, it should be remembered that the harder the cerebral palsied child tries to speak, the more unintelligible his speech often becomes. Nonspeaking children should be encouraged to give yes/no answers or communicate through their communication boards. Children with speech limitations should be given opportunities to participate in vocal activities such as songs and plays. Those unable to articulate can be taught to participate through body language, stamping their feet and raising their hands at appropriate times in the lyrics. A nonspeaking mainstreamed cerebral palsied fifth grader participated in the school play by using her foot to hit a switch which activated a tape recording of her part. She was thrilled to participate which was made possible because her teacher analyzed the problems and developed a workable solution.

Fatigue. For many with cerebral palsy, fatigue is a frequent problem. Often to accomplish even the most basic tasks tremendous effort has to be expended. The more severely handicapped who are placed in therapeutic equipment often spend long stretches of time in one position. A tired child is often irritable and unable to learn effectively. Watch for signs of fatigue and change the pace of the work. Reposition those who are in adaptive equipment.

Perceptual Problems. For those with cerebral palsy, learning is often uneven. Many tend to reach a plateau in their learning progress or show an understanding of one concept but have "strange gaps" in concepts that should have preceded. For example, a child may be able to count to 10 but have difficulty comprehending the meaning of size and spatial relationships. When asked to fill a glass from a pitcher, the child may overfill and become upset. He knew that 8 was bigger than 3 but yet could not see that the glass would not hold all the liquid from the pitcher. These learning inconsistencies are often referred to as perceptual learning disabilities.

Body Image. Some children with cerebral palsy have poorly developed body awareness. Often children with cerebral palsy have not had the same experiences with putting their bodies through space (spatial relationships) as other children. Finger games, rhymes, modeling bodies with clay, and songs may help these children become aware of their bodies and how each part relates to each other (DeChiara, 1980). Making patterns with bricks or beads is also helpful in developing the awareness of position in space. A prereading child will need instruction in such concepts as up/down, in/out, beside/under, and right/left.

Visual Constancy. Another field of perception in which a disability may lead to anxiety or a feeling of insecurity is visual constancy. If the shape, size, color, or brightness of a familiar object is changed, the child may not recognize it. For example, if a dog is drawn a little differently or a letter written in a different type, the child may not recognize it. Many children who have a tendency to perseverate may have visual constancy problems. This can cause significant reading delays (Weber, 1980). One way to help is to allow the child practice in handling the same object in different sizes, shapes, and colors.

Figure-Background. Figure-background relationships are often connected to visual constancy. The child will focus on an irrelevant object in the background. Distractibility may complicate this problem. The figure-background disturbance in perception can cause a child to be disorganized and inattentive.

Auditory. Some children have difficulty in processing information that is given auditorily—that is, they cannot remember the sequence of events in a story told orally or follow directions carefully. Practice in helping a child remember oral directions, number sequences, etc., is valuable. At first, visual cues may be necessary to aid the child.

All these factors—distractibility, perseveration, speech problems, fatigue, perceptual difficulties—impact greatly on the teaching methods employed. As has been emphasized previously, an individual approach must be taken with each child with cerebral palsy. Truly no two are alike!

General Curriculum Areas

Because of the wide diversity in intellectual functioning, not all cerebral palsied children will be able to learn to read, write, or do arithmetic. For those who function at a low cognitive level, these concepts will be too advanced; for others, the basics will be mastered quickly and reading will turn into literature, penmanship into essays, and arithmetic into calculus. Each child must have the opportunity to develop basic educational skills to the highest level he or she can attain. Innovative approaches will be required.

Arithmetic. The teaching of numbers is often impeded by the cerebral palsied child's lack of incidental, practical, and personal experiences. It is difficult for the child to relate to the value of a quarter if he has never held one or purchased anything. Establishing a school store may help the children gain practical knowledge and experience with numbers. Water play, measuring, building with bricks, and playing with different shapes also increase the child's first-hand knowledge of number, volume, weight, size, and order. An old-fashioned abacus is helpful. The effect of actually seeing and touching the beads is instructive in instilling number serialization and ordination.

Reading. When teaching a child with cerebral palsy to read, the goal will be the same as that for a normal child. It may be possible to instruct using the phonetic method for some children. However, for the language impaired, the sight approach is usually more productive. As with all children, it is helpful to use a personal approach in the classroom—a list of children's names, birthdays, and addresses; captions on art work; short stories. Lots of books should be available for the children to see. For children with problems turning pages, place a piece of tape on the edge of each page. This helps lift and separate pages and makes them easier to turn. Oral reading by the teacher widens the child's vocabulary, develops his imagination, and whets his interest.

Writing. Handwriting is often difficult for many cerebral palsied children to master. It can be a frustration for the hemiplegic as well as the athetoid. It is helpful to stick the sheet of paper down to prevent it from sliding. No cerebral palsied child should be given small lined paper before he is ready. Alternates to writing such as typing on an electric typewriter or a computer may need to be explored.

Teaching Methods

As has been noted, children with cerebral palsy have divergent learning styles. One child is able to accomplish the task as stated and is reinforced for his efforts by teacher praise; the other child needs more specific reinforcement and a different medium to convey the concept. Being able to modify an activity is the hallmark of good teaching. A curriculum enables a teacher to know *what* to teach, but a good teacher must also know *how* to teach it.

When teaching a cerebral palsied child, the experience should be success-oriented and provide reinforcement. Assisting the child in making the right response and then reinforcing his efforts will help ensure that the skill is acquired as quickly as possible. With children who are developing normally, it is sometimes beneficial to allow them to learn by trial and error. However, with handicapped children more structure is usually needed so that the child focuses on what response is expected and is correct.

Learning is enhanced through the child's active involvement with the concept. Multisensory experiences are important. If a child is learning animal names, it will be helpful for the child to *see* a picture of the animal, to hold or *touch* the animal model (or a real one if possible), to *hear* the name of the animal spoken, and to repeat or *say* the name itself. This approach of exposing the child to the same concept through many different senses increases the child's rate of learning.

It is often a major source of concern for teachers that skills that have been taught to a child are not retained but are "forgotten." It needs to be determined that a child can perform a task consistently. Overlearning is necessary in many instances to ensure memory retention. Practice, practice, and more practice is essential for handicapped children.

It is also important for the teacher to ensure that the skill the child has learned can be used in many settings. Often handicapped children acquire a new skill but are able to use it only in the place where it was learned. When a skill can be used only in an isolated or restricted setting (such as the classroom), it becomes nonfunctional because the object of teaching the skill in the first place was to make the child more independent. The child is not more independent if the only place he can accomplish his objective is at school. Therefore, the teacher needs to plan carefully for the child to transfer the learning to many different settings. The following is a list of instructional strategies that often help facilitate this transfer of learning.

1. Shift from primary to secondary reinforcers. Try to reinforce the child's efforts gradually using praise (secondary) rather than food (primary).
2. Thin out the schedule of reinforcers. Try giving a reinforcer every other time the child accomplishes the task rather than every time once he has shown he can do it; then decrease reinforcement to every third time, then occasionally, etc.
3. Train across a variety of language cues, people, and settings. Have the child wash his hands before lunch not only at school but when he is home over the weekend, or out to eat with the class at a restaurant, etc. Have him dry his hands with a paper towel one time, a cloth towel the next so that he can get used to different materials.
4. Reinforce the desired skill in a novel environment. Remember to praise the child for performing the objective in a place that he has not practiced it. When a setting is new to him, he may need more reinforcement to realize that the objective he now does automatically at school is important in the new environment, such as washing his hands, or communicating with a stranger.
5. Train adults in the various environments in which the child has contact. Be sure to let parents, day care workers, babysitters, and others know what they should do to encourage or reinforce the child's efforts.

Many teachers find that the curriculum they have chosen presents the objectives and activities for the children in steps that are often too large. For example, in a curriculum that was chosen by the teacher, the self-help objective appropriate for Elsie specified that "the child will put on the sock unassisted." However, when the teacher demonstrates the way to do this, Elsie finds it is just too difficult. Elsie learns more quickly when the objective is broken down into small, easily understood parts. Therefore, the teacher decides to employ task analysis. Task analysis is simply the breaking down of any objective into individual steps. These steps are then taught separately but in order.

There are two ways to break down an objective—forward chaining and backward chaining. Forward chaining is used when the teaching begins with the first step and proceeds to the last step in order. Backward chaining teaches the last step first.

Objective: Puts on sock unassisted.
Forward chaining analysis:

1. Child places toes in sock.
2. Child pulls sock over the entire foot, heel correct.
3. Child pulls sock over heel.
4. Child pulls sock over ankle.
5. Child pulls sock up calf.

Backward chaining analysis:

1. Child puts on sock when just above heel.
2. Child puts on sock when below heel.
3. Child puts on sock when toes started in.
4. Child puts on sock when handed to him.
5. Child puts on sock.

Backward chaining (also called backward shaping or reverse chaining) is a useful technique for teaching self-help skills. The child begins by learning to do independently the last step first. Therefore, he is always completing the task himself—a rewarding feeling. Forward chaining is more appropriate for other objectives.

The ability to think through an objective and break it down is essential when teaching handicapped children. It is the teacher's responsibility to structure the objectives so that the child can learn and succeed. Task analysis is one of the best tools a teacher has to ensure that learning will take place.

Another teaching strategy that is often helpful to teachers is called successive approximation. When using successive approximation, the teacher shapes the behavior she desires through systematic reinforcement of steps in the direction of the goal. For example, Randy, age 10, has limited speech. His speech therapist feels it is now appropriate for Randy to say "more" instead of merely vocalizing when he wishes additional juice or cookies. First she requires Randy to make the "m" sound if he wishes additional drink or food. Next he is required to say "mo" and finally she requires him to say "more" at the appropriate time. By reinforcing his efforts through each phase, the teacher lets Randy know she is pleased with his performance. When the teacher changes her expectations (from a sound to the "m" sound) the teacher models the correct response and reinforces only Randy's more specific sounds—that is, "m." Randy gradually is able to attain his objective through a series of attempts or approximations that the teacher and therapist felt were appropriate.

REFERENCES

Bush, M. (1980). Institutions for dependent and neglected children: Therapeutic option of choice or last resort. *American Journal of Orthopsychiatry, 50,* 239–255.

DeChiara, E. (1980). Modeling cookie people helps improve body image. *Arts and Activities, 80,* 40–41, 56–57.

Forness, S. (1977). A transition model for placement of handicapped children in regular and special classes. *Contemporary Education Psychology, 2,* 37–49.

Heron, T. F. (1978). Maintaining the mainstreamed child in the regular classroom: The decision-making process. *Journal of Learning Disabilities, 11,* 210–216.

Jones, R. L., Gottlieb, J., Guskin, S., & Yoshida, R. K. (1978). Evaluating mainstreaming programs: Models, caveats, considerations and guidelines. *Exceptional Children, 4*, 588–601.

Miller, T. L., & Switzky, H. N. (1978). The least restrictive alternative: Implications for service providers. *Journal of Special Education, 12*, 123.

Newberger, D. A. (1978). Situational socialization: An affective interaction component of the mainstreaming reintegrating construct. *Journal of Special Education, 12*, 113–121.

Smith, C. R. (1983). *Learning disabilities: The interaction of learner, task and setting.* Boston: Little Brown.

Vance, H. B. (1980). Attention deficits and learning disabilities. *Education and Treatment of Children, 3*, 153–160.

Weber, G. Y. (1980). Visual disabilities: Their identification and relationship with academic achievement. *Journal of Learning Disabilities, 13*, 301–305.

ADDITIONAL READINGS

Calhoun, M. L., & Hawisher, M. (1980). *Teaching and learning strategies for physically handicapped students.* Baltimore, MD: University Park Press.

Cruickshank, W. H. (1976). *Cerebral palsy: A developmental disability.* Syracuse, NY: Syracuse University Press.

EC:EEN Project. (1979). *Programmed training.* WI: Wisconsin Department of Public Instruction.

Fullagar, P. K., & Glover, M. E. (1977). *Competency based training for staff serving developmentally disabled children.* Durham, NC: Chapel Hill Training-Outreach.

Jordan, J., Hayden, A., Karnes, M., & Woods, M. M. (Eds.). (1977). *Early childhood education for exceptional children.* Reston, VA: The Council for Exceptional Children.

Mid-East Regional Resource Center. (1979). *Implementation of the individualized education program: A teacher's perspective.* Washington, DC: George Washington University.

Oswin, M. (1967). *Behavior problems amongst children with cerebral palsy.* Bristol: John Wright & Sons.

Stafford, P. L. (1978). *Teaching young children with special needs.* St. Louis, MO: C. V. Mosby.

United States Statutes at Large, 1975. (1977). Washington, DC: U.S. Government Printing Office.

Weiner, S. (1980). I'm not dumb, am I? How to help children with learning disabilities. *Childhood Education, 56*, 156–160.

CHAPTER 13

Advanced Technology Aids for Communication, Education, and Employment

Gregg C. Vanderheiden

Technology is playing an ever-increasing role in the lives of all people and has many applications in programs for persons disabled by cerebral palsy. Many factors must be considered when selecting an aid for a cerebral palsied individual, and it must be recognized that not all persons with cerebral palsy will be able to utilize "high tech" aids. The speech/language pathologist must be familiar with what high tech aids can— and cannot—do and be aware of adaptations which make aids accessible to persons with poor motor control.

1. *How does Vanderheiden distinguish between a* needs *and a* features *approach to selecting an aid?*
2. *For each of the five possible needs Vanderheiden describes, list what should be considered when assessing the need.*
3. *Discuss the strategies or adaptations which give persons with poor motor control greater access to information processing systems.*

INTRODUCTION

Advancing technology is providing new opportunities and new tools for individuals with severe physical handicaps. As our world becomes more automated, physical disability is becoming less handicapping. More and more jobs are centered around handling and processing information, rather than handling and processing objects. Naisbitt (1984) forecasts that by 1990, 75% of all jobs will involve computers in some way, and people who cannot use them will be at a disadvantage. Even our homes and daily lives are being increasingly automated. It is now possible to control a large number of appliances in our houses by remote control without relying on any special devices made specifically "for the disabled." Soon, banking and shopping will also be possible without leaving our homes. Even home-based employment is now being developed. As society moves in these directions, the disabled individual can spend less time in travel and caring for basic needs. More time will be available for creative activity, productive activity, and travel for social pursuits. In order to tap this potential, however, the disabled individual must be able to access and use various automated and information processing systems. This primary problem will be addressed later in this chapter.

At the same time that technology is making society more amenable to and accessible to individuals with physical disabilities, it is also providing new materials and tools to the rehabilitation personnel. Specifically developed communication, control, and writing aids are now available to disabled individuals which were not possible 10 years ago. In addition, the rapid advances of microcomputers, particularly portable microcomputers, is reducing the cost of many of these advanced aids. Further, these aids are beginning to be powerful enough to seriously address the problems of young children and individuals with language impairments.

These new technologies, however, also pose very real potential dangers. Because the aids spark our imaginations and seem to have so much power, they are often employed too early in an individual's communication program, or in the wrong fashion. In general, these technical aids are best used to overcome physical problems or physical limitations to communication. For that reason, advanced aids are most useful to individuals whose major barrier to communication is an inability to converse or write due to a physical handicap. Often, however, these aids are applied with individuals who are not yet communicating or interacting even with simpler systems. Individuals who are not communicating effectively on communication boards are often provided with advanced aids in the hope that the advanced aid will somehow instill communicative competence in the individual. This would be somewhat akin to providing someone with a grand piano because he is not playing well (or at all) on a spinet.

Thus, the early application of technology can confuse the issue and misdirect attention in the intervention program. Introduction of an aid before it is needed often puts the focus of the program on mastering the aid rather than on developing communicative competence and interactive behaviors. When this happens, technology misdirects and delays the child's development rather than advancing it. Understanding of what technology is and is not, what it can and cannot do, and a healthy skepticism about its usefulness is essential to its successful application. Clinicians and rehabilitation personnel must be careful that their fascination with technology and its potentials does not result in application of it where it is not useful, or too early in an intervention program.

THE NATURE OF COMMUNICATION AND CONTROL NEEDS

The best way to keep a proper perspective on technology is to approach it from a *needs* rather than a *features* point of view. A features approach generally focuses on the aids and what they can do. Such information must be considered when selecting an aid; however, features are important only when they can be employed by disabled persons to meet specific needs.

A needs approach, however, provides two functions. First, it turns our focus toward the particular needs of an individual at his current level of competency. For example, if we focus on interaction as our objective, and we try to focus or direct our attention toward what the individual needs, or what will assist in improving interaction within the environment, we often find that the needs are not technical in nature. More often than not, the needs are for a larger and more relevant vocabulary, more interaction time, a more interactive environment, and more meaningful communicative situations—not just situations where the message receivers ask questions to which they already know the answers.

The second advantage of a needs-oriented approach is that, where technology may be of benefit, the full range of the individual's needs can be profiled, and an aid which best matches *the entire range of needs* can be secured. For example, with a features approach one might recommend an aid with voice output and a programmable vocabulary, because both these features are useful for many individuals.

The needs approach emphasizes identifying not only the conversational needs of a client but also the writing and other needs. In the elementary grades, a cerebral palsied child would need an aid to handle pencil and paper tasks such as spelling and written assignments. In higher grades more extensive written work is required, including mathematics. In an increasing number of classrooms, computers are used for some assignments. To carry out these educational activities and to function well in this environment, the child would also need a visible, correctable display for mastering spelling and sentence construction; a multiple line display for doing mathematics problems; some form of printout to allow for such activities as independent work, worksheet completion, and testing; a mechanism for accessing the computers used by classmates in addition to a mechanism for conversation to handle questions and discussions and for social interaction. An aid with only voice output and programmable vocabulary features would neither meet nor address all of the client's needs—the client would be able to converse but would be unable to participate in the educational program. Furthermore, the cost of a voice-only aid is generally so high that it prohibits the acquisition of additional aids to meet the other needs of the client. When selecting an aid, the question is not whether the client could use a particular aid but whether it is the best aid to meet the full range of the client's needs, which includes: (a) conversation needs (and messaging), (b) writing needs (portable and workstation), (c) computer access needs, (d) access to control panels, and (e) manipulation needs.

Conversation Needs and Messaging

This is the most commonly thought of need when communication is first mentioned. In fact, in many cases it is treated synonymously with "communication."

With conversational needs, most of the focus has been on providing an individual with a "voice." However, *rate* is much more important than *form* for conversation (i.e., visual or vocal). Normal conversation takes place at the rate of about 180 words per minute (wpm). Conversation can be held at slower rates, but it is extremely difficult, if not impossible, to carry on a conversation in the usual sense of the word if the communication rate is limited to 2 to 8 wpm. This is especially true if one of the conversational parties is communicating at 180 wpm and the other is communicating at 2 to 8 wpm. Although communication and interaction can and do take place in such situations, the rules of normal conversation are violated, and interactions are generally short, dominated by one party, and highly frustrating to both. This is true whether the form of communication is written, visual, or spoken.

When the rates are more rapid, however, conversations can and do take place routinely in a wide variety of forms. Speech is by far the most common and fastest mode of conversation. However, effective conversation through signs and gestures is common, and conversations using typed media, telecommunication devices for the deaf (TDDs), and other visual and printed forms, routinely take place.

The lure of voice is so powerful, however, that most people identify voice with language, and make the erroneous assumption that if they can provide their client with a voice of some type, then the client will be able to "talk" and "converse." In fact, although voice output is indeed both powerful and desirable, communication rate is nevertheless a more important factor than form in the selection of an effective means of conversational communication.

With the current technology, it is not possible to produce the rates necessary for normal conversation. The average individual using an augmentative communication aid can communicate at a rate of approximately 3–5 wpm. With better prescription and therapies, it is possible to increase the rate to 10–15 wpm, which is far below the 180 wpm rate of normal conversation. In fact, the fastest mechanism for carrying on a conversation or interaction at the present time is to use a manual type of communication (manual scanning or manual pointing board), and allow the message receiver to construct sentences and concepts from cues given by the nonspeaking individual. A single letter or two is usually sufficient cue for the receiver to guess a word, and two or three words in a sentence frequently enable the receiver to guess the entire sentence accurately. By proceeding in this fashion, it is possible to communicate at a rate which is perhaps 5–8 times faster than the rate at which the individual would normally be able to communicate. Moreover, this type of anticipation and assistance is not possible with current technological communication aids; nor is it probable that these rates can be matched by such aids in the near future. Advanced forms of artificial intelligence which allow semantic construction based upon context and only limited cues from the handicapped individual will be required. We are only beginning to scratch the surface of this technology.

For a small percentage of those using augmentative communication, some new techniques may provide communication rates which approximate normal conversational rates. For the vast majority of individuals, however, nonautomated communication aids will remain the fastest methods for conversation. Some clients with automated communication boards, for example, turn off the aids and use them as manual pointing boards in general conversation. They turn the aid on only when they are with a stranger who is unfamiliar with the communication process or if they are with an uncooperative communicator who interrupts or will not let them finish their thoughts. Manual communication boards, however, cannot by themselves meet all the conversation needs of nonspeaking individuals. Manual boards are often ambiguous, require a trained message receiver, require the undivided attention of the receiver, do not allow interjection of quick conversational phrases, and do not allow for private or independent revision or extension of the vocabulary and phrases of the boards by the users. Thus, although at this time manual boards may be the most efficient approach, they are not always effective or sufficient when used alone.

In discussing conversation aids, a contrast is often made between the advantages of a visual and printed output form and a voice output form. Both have advantages, and, as we will see, a fully functional communication aid would have both a visual, correctable display and voice output. Voice output provides the child with the ability to interrupt, to continue his conversation even after the message receiver has diverted complete attention, to talk to people who are busy at other tasks (e.g., cooking, repairing something, cleaning, watching television); facilitates communicating with groups of individuals; and allows communication with younger, prereading individuals. The visible, correctable display has many advantages: (a) it provides communication with persons who might not understand the current voice output, (b) it enables the individual to use words he knows but cannot spell by allowing him to approximate spellings, (c) it is easier for other individuals to decipher poorly constructed or expressed sentences by giving them time to study the sentences visually to determine what the child means, (d) it allows the child to speed up communication by using contractions, skipping words, etc., which might make a spoken message undecipherable, and (e) it allows the child to meet the important need for written communication. Thus, it is not a question of voice *or* visual display output, but rather voice *and* visual display output. Where only one can be provided, however, the visual display with a printer is far superior to the voice-only aid for any child who has the potential of learning to spell or use printed words.

Technology is beginning to address conversational needs by providing low-cost visual correctable displays, printed output, and synthetic speech. Effective rate of communication, however, remains a major problem, as current technologies are only beginning to address this problem. At the present time, the best approaches for increasing rate are to provide optimal positioning and seating of the individual to allow control of faster communication techniques, and to develop better communication strategies which enable the individual to communicate more effectively.

Messaging is a technique used only occasionally by normal speakers, and then not as a form of conversation. Cerebral palsied persons with slow communication rates, however, use messaging much more extensively to meet needs usually handled through conversation. It is sometimes assumed that a slow communicator can carry on a conversation by simply preparing his message in advance, and presenting it to the message receiver at the appropriate time. But because the receiver's response cannot be anticipated, only the opening sentence of the conversation can be prepared in advance. As soon as the second party responds, the first party must communicate at his real time rate, which may be only 2–8 wpm. Thus, what results is usually not a "conversation," but rather an introduction of the topic by the handicapped individual, followed by an interaction dominated by the second party. Though messaging has limitations, it is still an effective procedure. It can also be used by handicapped individuals following the interaction to prepare rebuttals or follow-up comments which express their thoughts. Messaging is facilitated most if the individual's communication aid has some form of printed output. Current technologies are good to excellent in meeting this communication need. Aids which have sufficient memory can also be used in this fashion with only visual or voice output. Without a printout, however, many of the normal messaging uses are eliminated, and the aid is limited to functioning as a "conversation starter." Fortunately, the advent of pocket computers and printing calculators is bringing the cost of miniature printers down, and making the provision of portable printed output much easier than it was in even the recent past.

Writing Needs

The communication needs of a cerebral palsied individual do not end with conversation. Written communication abilities are required for most education, vocational, or productive activities.

Portable Writing Needs. Normally developing children find it necessary to write in performing a variety of educational tasks in a variety of places, such as completing written exercises in school or at home. Pencil and paper are standard, portable, and essential student educational materials, but cerebral palsied children with poor arm and hand function may not be able to use pencil and paper. They need special aids for tasks such as taking notes, completing worksheets, or writing themes. While useful for children with cerebral palsy, a typewriter, even when equipped with expanded keyboard or special keyguards, cannot meet all the writing needs of the physically handicapped individual. A personal, portable means of writing is essential in order to provide the physically handicapped individual with a reasonable chance for education or employment. This means of writing must be available at all times to these individuals in the same manner that the normal child has access to a pencil and paper.

To perform functions similar to those usually performed with pencil and paper, a writing aid must have several characteristics:

1. It is critical that the aid perform at an acceptable rate. Providing handicapped individuals with a means of writing which is 5 to 10 times slower than that of other children will prevent them from keeping up with the output of handicapped peers. The ability to com-

plete one day's work every week or two is unacceptable in education or employment, and severely retards or reduces the individual's development.

2. Both a visual correctable display and some type of printed output are essential.

3. A multiple-line rather than a single-line display is especially important for those who will be using the aid to develop their basic writing and math skills. At least four lines of display are necessary to allow the individual to arrange math problems in the traditional format so they are easier to understand and solve. Adding two numbers written side by side (e.g., "345 + 674 = ?"), as would be required on a single line display, is difficult, especially for those who are just beginning to develop math skills.

Equipment is being developed to address the problems of display and rate. Portable microcomputers are available with multiple-line displays and built-in printers. These microcomputers can be used as the core of specially designed communication/control aids for more severely physically handicapped individuals.

Compared to conversation needs, writing needs are much easier to address. Matching the normal written rate of 30–35 wpm is much easier than matching the conversational rate of 180 wpm. Individuals who can produce 5–10 wpm can "write" at one-third the normal rate. Some newer techniques can double or triple the individual's rate of straight typing, bringing this 5–10 wpm up to the normal rate of handwriting. The more severely involved individuals may not be able to achieve this handwriting rate. However, their rate of communication will always be about six times closer to the writing rate than to the conversation rate of their peers. A more rapid rate of communication will be helpful both in education and in some types of employment, where performance is more a function of thinking and writing than of conversation.

Workstation Writing Needs. Though workstation writing needs are similar to the portable writing needs, they are discussed separately because some large writing tasks might better be handled on a stationary writing system. At the present time, it is possible to provide more power and better display options in stationary systems than are currently possible in portable systems. This is changing rapidly, however, and full-scale workstations are already beginning to appear which are no larger than a three-ring notebook.

It is important to differentiate those tasks that can be handled in stationary writing situations from those that *must* be met by a portable aid. Because of the greater capabilities provided by stationary writing systems, there is a tendency to secure stationary systems for individuals who, in fact, have a greater need for portable systems. In general, the portable system is needed first, with a stationary system being provided for those individuals with sufficient writing needs that they require both. Eventually, the stationary system will become unnecessary or will take the form of expansions to the portable system. This transition may be technically feasible in a few years but will probably depend on the development of appropriate specialized software.

Access to Computers and Information Processing Systems

This need is less obvious to those whose education preceded the widespread use of computers and whose workplaces are untouched or barely touched by computers today. The use of computers in both education and employment, however, is increasing at an extremely rapid rate, and physically handicapped children who are unable to access and use the computers available to their classmates will be at a severe disadvantage and will be unable to participate in many of the educational activities in future classrooms. Of particular concern are those physically handicapped individuals who might develop their cognitive abilities to compensate for their lower physical skills. In employment situations, the inability to access and use computers will be an even greater handicap, especially for those individuals who will be making their livings using their minds. The ability to use computers can greatly facilitate many activities which are currently difficult for physically handicapped individuals to accomplish. As the business world and society in general move toward electronic information processing, more activities will be available which do not require normal physical manipulation skills—hence the physical manipulation problems of persons with cerebral palsy will become less handicapping. Their ability to fit into the socioeconomic world will improve through the use of these information and data processing systems.

Computer access may be viewed as a communication task, similar to the problem of conducting a conversation with another person using a communication aid. Both involve the transfer of information through a special keyboard or interface of some type. The techniques, interfaces, and aids necessary to provide this interface to the computer are similar, if not identical, to those required for conversation. In a later section of this chapter, the need for developing accessing skills will be discussed further, and solution strategies for providing access to standard computers will be presented.

Access to Controls and Control Panels Needed for Daily Living

Use of an environmental control system can greatly enrich the quality of life for persons with cerebral palsy. Technology is available by which persons with severe physical handicaps can operate radios, television, lights, doors, telephones, information systems, climate control systems, and mobility systems.

Handicapped individuals often have a need to communicate with or operate the non-keyboard devices which are part of environmental control systems. This includes control panels as well as general environmental device control. At the present time, environmental control systems are largely separate from an individual's communication system; however, the trend is toward integration of these systems.

Manipulation

Robots today are found primarily in industrial applications. Eventually robots and other remote manipulators will come into more general use. We can speculate that in the future it will be possible to have robots carry out many of the manipulative functions required by a physically handicapped individual. However, advances in environmental control and robotics will be of little use to an individual who cannot communicate with or control these devices. When general-purpose, mobile, multifunctional robots become a reality, the disabled person's communication and control system must be able to provide them with a way to access them.

STRATEGIES FOR ACCESS TO COMPUTERS AND INFORMATION PROCESSING SYSTEMS

One of the most powerful advanced technologies is the microcomputer; however, there is considerable confusion about how it might be used in the rehabilitation process. This confusion stems in part from a lack of understanding of what the computer is. Another source of confusion stems from the fact that microcomputers can play a variety of roles in the lives of disabled individuals.

What a Computer Is and Isn't

A computer is a simple, yet flexible device which is basically nothing more than *a machine which carries out instructions.* By itself a computer doesn't add, subtract, think, or word process. It simply follows instructions contained in a computer program. While computers can carry out these instructions accurately and quickly, the tremendous accomplishments which have been attributed to computers should be attributed directly to the programs, not the computer. It is the program (i.e., the instructions) that causes the computer to act like a word processor, a calculator, a communication aid, a tutor, a chemistry lab, or a specialized aid for disabled children. If we are confused because the computer does not seem to act the same all the time, it is because we think the computer "acts" at all.

In fact, it is the "software" or programs which do all of the acting. Change the program (the instructions) for a computer, and it will behave differently.

With this understanding, it is easy to answer the question of what a computer can and cannot do. A computer can do anything for which someone can write a precise set of instructions in the computer's machine language and which the computer is physically capable of doing. For example, a computer can't provide a print-out if a printer is not connected. Neither can a computer solve a problem that no one knows how to solve because no one would be able to write the instructions for the computer to follow. It is inappropriate to consider computers as smart or intelligent. They are machines which function as slaves precisely following the instructions given to them. Of course, to solve more complex problems, more complex programs must be written and more powerful computers are needed to carry out the instructions. Regardless of the "power" of a computer it is the "software," i.e., programs, which determine how useful the computer will be to individuals with disabilities.

The Roles of Computers With Disabled Persons

Not all persons with cerebral palsy will be able to utilize computers, but for those with sufficient cognitive development, computers might be used in two ways (Bowe, 1984; McWilliams, 1984; Vanderheiden, 1982). First, they could be used as a special device which follows instructions tailored to fit the needs of disabled persons. For example, in this role a computer, using an appropriate program, could function as a communication aid or it might be set up as a one-switch scanning device to present a computerized reading program. In a second role, the computer would perform the same functions as it does for nondisabled persons and use the same programs. This role is ever-growing in scope and importance. The following list suggests some ways in which many persons with cerebral palsy will use computers: (a) mechanisms for communication, (b) writing systems, (c) to accelerate speed of keyboard use, (d) filing and transmitting information, (e) accessing information, (f) conducting financial transactions, and (g) making precision drawings.

Using appropriate programs, computers can provide additional educational opportunities for persons with cerebral palsy—even enabling them to carry out experiments in chemistry, physics, and other sciences involving manipulations that they would otherwise be unable to perform. Computers can make it possible for many disabled persons to live alone by providing them with monitoring systems which can be programmed to detect environmental changes or an *absence* of daily living activities, which then automatically triggers a call for assistance.

Disabled persons will also use computers for the same purposes as nondisabled persons. As our society increasingly utilizes computer systems in educational, business, banking, recreational—in fact, most activities—any individual who is unable to access and use these systems will be at an extreme disadvantage. It is essential that persons with cerebral palsy be provided with more than just the programs designed specifically for them. They must be able to access and use standard computers and programs as they find them in their communities, shopping centers, schools, and workplaces.

Barriers to Computer Use by Disabled Individuals

The principal barrier to use of computers by cerebral palsied individuals is a physical inability to operate the standard keyboard-type input mechanisms. Some individuals can use keyboards with special keyguards on them but are unable to hold down multiple keys as is sometimes required. Other individuals are totally unable to use a keyboard. Development of new input techniques such as touchscreens, voice input, lightpens, and touchpads may enable many persons with poor arm and hand control to access the computer, but will provide additional barriers to others.

In addition to the physical access problem, many individuals with cerebral palsy also have visual problems to varying degrees. The original TV-based video displays on computers provided fairly legible output and the display could be enlarged by using special or larger TV screens. Newer systems, however, use smaller and more finely detailed video displays. In addition, many computer companies have replaced the large letters, located in the center of each key on the keyboard, with small letters positioned in the upper corners of the keys. While more stylish, these key letters are often difficult or impossible to read for individuals with visual disabilities, or for those who have keyguards mounted on their keyboards.

Adaptations to Provide Access

To address this problem, special programs have been written for disabled individuals which do not require the use of the standard keyboards. Many of these are described in *Communication, Control, and Computer Access for Disabled and Elderly Individuals* (Brandenburg & Vanderheiden, 1986). For example, programs have been written using scanning techniques which require only a single switch. Knee, hand, shoulder, tongue, breath, and even eyegaze can be used to control these programs. Other special programs have been written which use two-switch Morse code, joysticks, optical beams attached to the head, etc., as input modes. These are special programs written specifically for disabled individuals. They do not address the important problem of providing access to all of the standard software and the multitude of other computers that the disabled individual will encounter in his education, vocational, and daily living environments.

Access Strategies for Standard Software.   To have access to standard computer systems, the disabled person will need some type of "transparent" access techniques that access the computer in such a way that the computer *cannot perceive—in any way—that it is not being used in a normal fashion*. For example, a severely disabled person, using a transparent access mechanism, would be able to enter information into the computer using just his eyegaze, and the computer would be unable to tell that the individual was not typing on its keyboard with his fingers in the same fashion as anyone else. Because the effect would be the same as typing directly on the keyboard, the person would be able to run any standard, off-the-shelf software that used the keyboard for input, without having to modify the software in any way. Similarly, the person would be able to run software on any computer for which he had a transparent access mechanism.

A simple example of a transparent access mechanism is the computer keyguard. Those who are unable to use a standard keyboard may be able to type using a keyguard—a plate mounted above the keyboard. Holes in the keyguard over each key guide the finger to the desired key and prevent it from touching other keys. Special latching mechanisms fitted onto the keyguard over the SHIFT, CONTROL, and ALTERNATE keys may be used to lock one of those keys down. The hand is then free to strike a second key, as would be required to shift from a lower case to a capital letter, for example. The computer (and its software program) would not be able to tell that the individual was not depressing both keys himself, per the original design.

A more powerful transparent access mechanism is the Keyboard Emulating Interface (KEI) (Kelso & Gunderson, 1984; Vanderheiden, 1982). This interface makes keyboards accessible to many disabled individuals who can't use standard keyboards. Figure 13.1A shows a computer and its keyboard. Normally, as a person types on the keyboard, electronic signals are sent to the computer telling the computer which keys are being depressed. The KEI is a small electronic module which creates the same electrical signals as the keyboard. The user unplugs the standard keyboard, and plugs in the KEI where the keyboard was, then plugs the standard keyboard back into the KEI. The KEI will accept signals from either the standard keyboard or a special aid, and send the signals into the computer in such a way that they look exactly like the signals that come from the keyboard (Figure 13.1B). Because the signals generated by the KEI are exactly the same as those generated by the keyboard, the computer is unable to tell that these "keystrokes" are not coming from the keyboard. Other special communication or interface aids can be plugged into the KEI. These aids could be operated by sip-and-puff, a single switch, eyegaze, or any other approach which best matches the individual user (see Figure 13.1C). Because the keyboard emulating interface is transparent, it does not affect the use of the computer by non-disabled persons at all. Even with the KEI in place, the computer and its

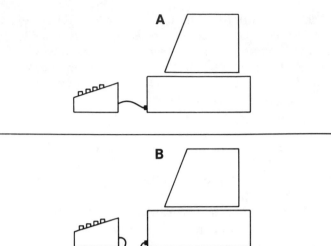

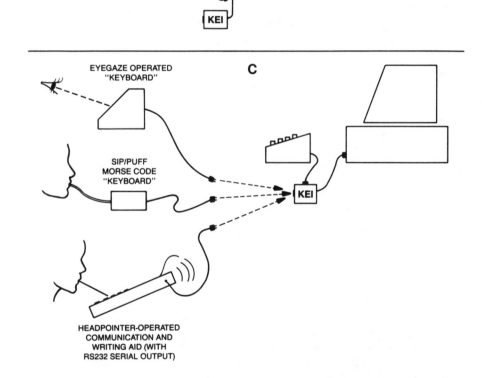

Figure 13.1. A. Computer with its normal keyboard. B. Computer with Keyboard Emulating Interface connected where keyboard used to be. C. Computer with Keyboard Emulating Interface allows use by individuals using a wide range of input techniques.

normal keyboard would function precisely as it did before the interface was installed.

Other Solution Strategies and Future Problems. Keyboard emulating interfaces, however, do not solve the entire problem. Computers are being developed with input methods designed to take increased advantage of the physical capabilities of nonhandicapped individuals. For example, input techniques such as "mice," body tracking systems, touchscreens, and voice input may make computer access easier for able-bodied individuals but more difficult for individuals with severe physical and communication handicaps. Transparent access methods for computers using these specialized input techniques are also under development, and the possibility of programming software solutions to these access problems is being explored. This strategy would involve changing the instructions inside the standard computers so that they allow access from both the standard keyboard and alternate input techniques. Unfortunately, the operating systems and software in the current computers, particularly the low-cost computers, do not support this strategy. The problem is further complicated by the fact that computers and operating systems are changing rapidly; hence, any software "patch" or "fix" soon becomes obsolete as a new version of the operating system and software appears. Work is proceeding, however, in cooperation with the manufacturers of standard computers, to determine whether such alternate input strategies can be provided as a part of the standard software and operating systems as they are manufactured.

SUMMARY AND CONCLUSIONS

Aids using advanced technology can be powerful tools for assisting in communication, education, and employment for persons with severe physical handicaps. Their effectiveness, however, is dependent upon proper application, which in turn depends upon a thorough understanding of the potentials and limitations of these technical aids. One common mistake is to focus on the aids themselves, and their features, rather than focusing on the total needs of the individual. When considering communication and control aids, it is important to look at all of the communication and control needs of the individual—their conversational needs, writing needs, and need to access to standard computers and computer systems.

A new and powerful advance in technology has been the development of the microcomputer. This device can be a powerful and flexible tool for handicapped individuals. However, it was not developed for handicapped individuals; it was developed for nondisabled individuals and is rapidly being incorporated into all aspects of our lives. Over the next 10 to 15 years, the microcomputer will be incorporated into our society in such a way that anybody who is unable to use standard computers and standard software packages will be excluded from many important activities of our society including recreation, education, and employment. For this reason, it is essential that we begin attending to the problem of access to standard software and standard computer systems for our disabled clients. Transparent interface techniques, such as the keyboard emulating interface, hold the best promise for providing this unrestricted access to standard software without interfering in any way with the standard operation of the computer by nondisabled individuals. Newer interface technologies such as touchscreens and "mice," however, will continue to provide challenges.

Advancing technology is thus providing both new tools and new problems. If, however, the access problems can be addressed, the information- and technology-based societies should make it easier for individuals with physical handicaps to live, learn, and be productive.

REFERENCES

Bowe, F. (1984). *Personal computers and special needs.* Berkeley, CA: Sybex Computer Books.

Brandenburg, S., and Vanderheiden, G. (1986). *Communication, Control, and Computer Access for Disabled and Elderly Individuals.* San Diego, CA: College-Hill Press.

Kelso, D. P., & Gunderson, J. (1984). Generic keyboard emulator architecture for transparent access to standard software by handicapped individuals. *Proceedings of the Second International Conference of Rehabilitation Engineering,* (pp. 50–51). Ottawa, Canada.

McWilliams, P. (1984). *Personal computers and the disabled.* New York: Doubleday.

Naisbitt, J. (1984). *Megatrends.* New York: Warner Books.

Vanderheiden, G. C. (1982). Computers can play a dual role. *BYTE, 7,* 136–162.

ADDITIONAL READINGS

Dahmke, M. (Ed.). (1982). *BYTE, 7*(9), entire issue.

Hoffman, P. (1984). *Proceedings of the Discovery 1984 Conference.*

Roehl, J. (Ed.). (1983). *Proceedings of Discovery 1983: Computers for the Disabled,* (entire volume).

Seaborn, T. (Ed.). (1981). Computing and the handicapped. *Computer, 14*(1), (entire volume).

Vanderheiden, G. C. (1983). Non-conversational communication technology needs of individuals with handicaps. *Rehabilitation World, 7,* 8–12.

Vanderheiden, G. C. (1983). Curbcuts and computers: Providing access to computers and information systems for disabled adults (Keynote Speech). *Computers for the Disabled Conference.* Minneapolis, MN.

OTHER SOURCES OF CONTINUING INFORMATION ON THE FIELD

Trace Center Reprint Service
Waisman Center
1500 Highland Avenue
Madison, WI 53705

Closing the Gap (a newspaper on computers and the disabled)
Budd Hagen, Editor
Route 2
Henderson, MN 56002

Communication Outlook
Artificial Language Laboratory
Michigan State University
East Lansing, MI 48824

COPH Bulletin
Congress on the Physically Handicapped
101 Irving Park Road
Rockford, IL 61102

APPENDIX: Individually Administered Tests Useable in Whole or in Part with CP Children and Adolescents

Name and Publisher	Areas Assessed	Level of Assessment	Age Level	Administered by	Time (min.)	Norm or Criterion	Comments
AAMD Adaptive Behavior Scale-Public School Version: American Association of Mental Deficiency	Adaptive behavior	Diagnosis Evaluation	6-12	Teacher Specialist Psychologist	15-30	N	Observations of behavior and interviews. Norms based on CA students in regular and special classes. Reliability and validity estimates based on use of clinical (not school) version. Ratings vary from rater to rater.
Alpern-Boll Developmental Profile, 2nd ed.: Western Psychological Services	Physical, self-help, academic, & communication	Screening Diagnosis	0-12	Specialist Psychologist		N	Structured interview with parents in 5 domains. Well standardized.
Assessment of Children's Language Comprehension: Consulting Psychologists Press	Receptive language	Screening	3-7	Specialist Psychologist	10-15	C	Small standardization sample and low reliability. A developmental inventory providing a qualitative assessment in both English and Spanish. Pointing response format.
Auditory Discrimination Test: Western Psychological Services	Auditory discrimination Memory	Screening	5-8	Teacher Specialist Psychologist	10-15	N	Yes-no response required. Child must understand concept of same/different. Not suitable for bilingual or non standard English.

Instrument	Characteristic Measured	Purpose	Age Range	Examiner	Time (min.)	N/C	Comments
Bayley Scales of Infant Development: Psychological Corp.	Mental Ability Motor Social	Diagnosis	0–3	Psychologist	45	N	Motor scale should not be used with CPs. Many items in the mental scale require motor responses and are not suitable for use with CPs. Best use is as downward extension of Binet for TMRs. Good norms and longitudinal studies.
Behavior Problem Checklist: Herbert C. Quay and D.R. Peterson, authors	Personality (over/under-reaction)	Screening	6–12	Teacher (or adult well acquainted with child)	15	C N	Teacher observes behavior. Interrater and other reliabilities in .60–.90 range. Results can provide information about individual differences in behavior. Norms from author.
Boehm Test of Basic Concepts: Psychological Corp.	School readiness	Screening Instructional Planning	3–9	Parent Teacher Specialist Psychologist	30–40	C N	Tests preschool and primary level concepts. Child points to picture to answer query. Low reliability. Validity data incomplete.
Bristol Social Adjustment Guide: Educational Industrial Testing	Behavioral disturbance (Hostility, peer maladaptiveness under-reaction.)	Screening Evaluation	5–16	Teacher	15	C	Teachers check presence or absence of positive and negative behaviors. Subscales have low validity. Norms should *not* be used.

Name and Publisher	Areas Assessed	Level of Assessment	Age Level	Administered by	Time (min.)	Norm or Criterion	Comments
BRP–*Behavior Rating Profile*: PRO-ED	Student, teacher, and parent scales and sociogram	Screening	6–18	Parent Teacher Specialist	30	N	Scales may be used separately or in conjunction with other components to identify students who may have problems, settings in which problems are prominent, and individuals with differing perceptions of the behavior or student.
Cain-Levine Social Competence Scale: Consulting Psychologists' Press	Adaptive behavior of TMRs	Diagnosis Planning	6–12	Teacher Specialist Psychologist	15–20	N	Observation of behavior. Scoring procedures are subjective.
Coloured Progressive Matrices: Psychological Corporation	General mental ability Visual special perception	Screening	5–12 (Other forms for older subjects.)	Specialist Psychologist	10	N	Nonverbal. Should be used with vocabulary test. No standardization data for U.S. Gestural or pointing response format.
DAB–*Diagnostic Achievement Battery*: PRO-ED	Listening, Speaking, Reading, Writing, & Math Components	Evaluation Planning	6–14	Teacher Specialist Psychologist	40–56	N	A series of achievement subtest , three of which may be given to groups, but many cannot be given as standardized to severely physically handicapped.

Name	Domain	Purpose	Age	Administrator	Time	Code	Comments
DTLA-2–Detroit Tests of Learning Aptitude: PRO-ED	Linguistic, Cognitive, Attention, & Motor Domains	Diagnosis	6-17	Specialist Psychologist	60-90	N	Two subtests in each domain, but not all of the 11 subtests can be used with severely handicapped persons. Subtests have good internal consistency and fair stability coefficients.
Gordon Occupational-Checklist: Psychological Corporation	Vocational interests	Planning	Adolescence	Teacher Specialist	20-25	N	Responses relate to categories found in the Dictionary of Occupational Titles. Useful tool for vocational exploration. Other measures needed for adequate educational programming. Checklist limited to jobs not requiring college education. Subject responds by writing.
Haeussermann Educational Evaluation: Manual by Grune Stratton	Cognitive	Planning Evaluation	2-6	Psychologist	60	C	Structured interview with suggestion for methodical modification depending on child's functional deficits. Requires neither manipulation nor speech.
Hiskey Nebraska Test of Learning Aptitude: Marshall Hiskey, author	Learning ability of hearing impaired and nonimpaired	Diagnosis Planning	3-17	Psychologist	45-75	N	A performance scale; some subtests require fine motor coordination but can be omitted. Others require pointing/gesturing. Strong correlation with Binet, Wechsler. Separate norms for hearing normal and hearing impaired. Most subtests cannot be used with severely involved.

Name and Publisher	Areas Assessed	Level of Assessment	Age Level	Administered by	Time (min.)	Norm or Criterion	Comments
Kaufman Assessment Battery for Children: American Guidance Services	General mental abilities Achievement	Diagnosis Evaluation	3–12	Psychologist	60	N	Promotional activity at time of publication over interpreted data on differences between and importance of division of scores into simultaneous and sequential processing.
KeyMath Diagnostic Arithmetic: American Guidance Services	Arithmetic	Diagnosis Planning Evaluation	5–11	Teacher Specialist Psychologist	30	N C	No upper age limit for remedial use. Good curriculum content validity. Appendix helps user translate results to behavioral objectives. Oral, pointing, and some writing in response format.
Keystone Visual Skills Test: Division of Mast Development Co.	Visual acuity	Screening	6–18	Specialist	5	N	Requires a verbalized response. Preschool form available for CA2-6.
Learning Accomplishment Profile: Chapel Hill (NC) Training Outreach Project Kaplan Press	Language, coordination, personal-social readiness	Diagnosis Evaluation	0–6	Teacher Specialist Psychologist	Var	C	Linked to the LAP curriculum.

Test/Publisher	Area	Purpose	Age	Administrator	Time	Code	Comments
Leiter International Performance Scale: Stoelting, Co.	General mental abilities	Diagnosis Evaluation	3–12	Psychologist	30–30	N	No verbal response required; instructions pantomimed. Useable with hearing impaired. Inadequate technical data but has survived test of time. Ability to move 1-inch square blocks required.
Minnesota Multiphasic Personality Inventory: Psychological Corporation	Personality	Diagnosis	18–adult	Psychologist	45–90	N	Can be administered to groups. Usually requires reading and marking answers, but can be adapted. Tapes available for visually impaired. Useful in defining adult personality charateristics. Subject responds by writing or sorting cards.
Ordinal Scales of Psychological Development: University of Illinois Press	Six levels of sensorimotor period	Screening	2 wks–2 yrs	Psychologist	Var	C	Experimental scale based on concepts of Piaget. No norms available. Data available from children of grad students and faculty at a state university. Research on environment indicates significant effects on attainment.
Peabody Individual Achievement: American Guidance Services	Reading Spelling Arithmetic	Diagnosis Evaluation	6–21	Teacher Specialist Psychologist	30–40	N	Can be used to determine which level of a narrow band test to use for more comprehensive information. Oral and pointing response format.

Name and Publisher	Areas Assessed	Level of Assessment	Age Level	Administered by	Time (min.)	Norm or Criterion	Comments
Peabody Picture Vocabulary Test Revised: American Guidance Services	Receptive vocabulary	Screening	2½–adult	Paraprofessional Teacher Specialist Psychologist	15	N	Low reliability. Words empirically selected. Use of IQ misleading. Not to be used in place of intelligence test. Subject responds by pointing or orally.
Pictorial Test of Intelligence: Riverside	General mental ability	Diagnosis Evaluation	3–8	Psychologist	45	N	Neither verbal nor manipulative response required. Answers far enough apart to allow response by looking at answer. Normed on representative sample of U.S. Correlates well with Binet, Wechsler.
Piers-Harris Children's Self Concept Scale: Counselor Recordings and Tests	Self concept	Screening	9–21	Teacher Specialist	15–20	N	Can be administered to groups. Usually requires marking answers but can be adapted.
Roswell-Chall Diagnostic Reading Test of Word Analysis Skills: Essay Press	Reading Word analysis	Screening Planning Evaluation	6–9	Teacher Specialist Psychologist	10	C N	Small standardization sample; useful in informal analysis. Oral and written response format.

Test/Source	Area	Purpose	Age	Administrator	Time	N/C	Comments
Social & Prevocational Information Battery: CTB-McGraw Hill	Living skills	Planning Evaluation	12–18	Teacher Specialist Psychologist	130–190	N C	Standardized on 1800 junior/senior high school EMR students in Oregon. Low reliability. Useful for placement decisions regarding community living arrangements, sheltered workshops. Orally administered. Another form (SP 1B-T) available for moderately retarded.
Stanford Binet Intelligence Scale: Riverside Press	General mental ability	Diagnosis Evaluation	3–18	Psychologist	30–40	N	Requires speech and manipulation ability. Useable with mildly physically disabled. Well established content validity results in its use as benchmark for other tests.
Stanford Diagnostic Reading: Psychological Corp.	Reading	Diagnosis Planning Evaluation	6–21	Teacher Specialist Psychologist	90–150	N C	Good standardization; several portions can be adapted for use by severely physically handicapped. Some pages too crowded. Multiple choice response format.
Test for Auditory Comprehension of Language: Developmental Learning Materials	Receptive language in English and Spanish	Diagnosis Evaluation	3–6	Specialist Psychologist	10–20	N	Small standardization sample. Useful with nonverbal children and those with speech and language difficulties. Pointing response used.

Name and Publisher	Areas Assessed	Level of Assessment	Age Level	Adminis-tered by	Time (min.)	Norm or Criterion	Comments
Tests for Everyday Living; Publishers Test Service	Living skills	Diagnosis Planning	12–18	Teacher Specialist	180	C	No national norms available. Low reliabilities. Useful with low-achieving high school students for career/consumer education. Subject responds by pointing.
TOLD–Test of Language Development: PRO-ED	Spoken language	Diagnosis	Pri-mary 4-0-8-11 Inter-mediate 8-6-12-11	Specialist	40		Seven subtests to measure different components of spoken language. Separate forms for primary.
TONI–Test of Non-verbal Intelligence: PRO-ED	Language-free measure of intelligence & reasoning	Screening	5–adult	Specialist Psychologist	20–30	N	Abstract problem solving tasks of increasing complexity. Examiner pantomimes instructions. Subjects point to answer but do not read, write or verbalize.
Wechsler Intelligence Scale for Children–Revised: Psychological Corporation	General verbal mental ability	Diagnosis Evaluation	6–16+	Psychologist	60	N	Only the verbal test should be used. Oral responses required. Much research supports use. (Not useful for trainables) Norms and procedures for hearing impaired available. Other forms available for children

Wide Range Achievement Test: Jastak Associates	Reading Arithmetic Spelling	Screening	6–21	Teacher Specialist Psychologist	15–25	N	Large print and Braille editions available also. Reading measured only by letter and word recognition which must be pronounced. Copying and writing required.
Woodcock–Johnson Psycho-Educational Battery: Teaching Resourses	Achievement Interest	Diagnosis Planning Evaluation	3–21	Psychologist	120	N	Oral and written responses. 27 subtests in 3 clusters. Good standardization measures and broad range of achievement.
Woodcock Reading Mastery: American Guidance Service	Reading	Diagnosis Planning Evaluation	6–18	Teacher Specialist Psychologist	40	N C	Large standardization sample. Excellent for use with students with reading problems. Oral response; training needed for interpretation.

None of the tests are useable with all cerebral palsied children. Most require some adaptations which may cause validity to be questioned. Additional information about the tests can be found in:

Bagnato, S. J., & Neisworth, J. T., 1981. *Linking developmental assessment and curricula.* Rockville, MD: Aspen Publications.

Lambert, N. (Ed.). 1981. *Special Education Assessment Matrix.* Monterey, CA: CTB McGraw Hill.

Mitchell, J. B. (Ed.). 1985. *The ninth mental measurements yearbook.* Lincoln, NE: The University of Nebraska Press.

Author Index

Subject Index